The Art of
Being Beautiful

Bedford Shelmire, Jr., M.D.

The Art of
Being Beautiful

ST. MARTIN'S PRESS, NEW YORK

Contents

I Prospectus

There are no beauty secrets, only beauty facts that women either don't know or don't fully understand. The one and only key to a more beautiful appearance is having the right information, and then putting it to practical use.

Unfortunately, accurate and reliable beauty information isn't always easy to get. Women are continually being told by someone or other what they must do to be beautiful, but much of this advice is based on bad information. It comes from well-meaning friends and from those who provide various services, such as beauticians, cosmetic salespeople, and cosmetologists; it comes in a never-ending stream from radios, television sets, newspapers, and magazines. Even the most cursory reference to any of these sources will instantly confirm the fact that all the old myths and half-truths are not only alive, but flourishing. Women are still told that their skin "breathes," that it can be "nourished" with something that comes out of a jar, and that their pores can be opened and closed as easily as their refrigerator doors. Some of this misinformation is the result of honest ignorance, but much of it is generated by people who are trying to sell something. If a particular product or service lacks effectiveness, which is often the case, its promoters must rely on deceptive or misleading advertising to generate sales. The conflicts and contradictions inherent in all this bad advice are perfectly obvious, so it is no wonder that most women are confused, skeptical, and unsure of themselves as far as personal beauty care is concerned.

In the belief that this situation could be remedied to some extent, I recently wrote a book called *The Art of Looking Younger.* In it I tried to point out that many of the visible changes we associate with age are due to neglect and abuse, rather than heredity. I tried to tell readers how these aging changes might be avoided with proper care, and not only explained the specific details of various methods, but recommended products by brand name. The present book is a continuation of these efforts to provide concise and useful beauty information, and to help women achieve their maximum potential with a minimum of time, effort, and expenditure. It is, however, considerably broader in scope than the earlier book. This approach was dictated by the fact that beauty needs change from year to year, and each age is subject to certain unique problems that call for individual attention.

This book begins with infancy, where beauty care should begin, and goes on to examine the beauty needs and beauty problems encountered at each stage of life. It will tell you which specific products and methods are most effective in meeting these needs and solving these problems. It will discuss not only the complexion and figure, but the hair, nails, hands, feet, and every other part of the body that is seen by anyone at any time. In short, the object of this book is to present a comprehensive guide to the care of the total appearance throughout life.

First we will cover the basic principles of beauty care.

These are all very simple and easy to understand, and you will be better equipped to carry out your personal beauty routine if you know beforehand what you are trying to accomplish. Following this are the chapters giving the details of beauty care for each age group, covering both routine beauty care and special beauty problems. Chapters V through VIII are keyed to biological rather than chronological age, and determining your Personal Skin Index will indicate which of these chapters is most applicable to you. Instructions for doing this are given in Chapter IV. With your PSI as a guide, you can be sure of finding the specific beauty routine, and the products and services, that will work best for you.

The products recommended in this book are all simple, inexpensive, and easily obtainable at supermarkets, drugstores, and variety stores. These recommendations are not based on price alone, but on the fact that simple and inexpensive beauty aids often work better, and are safer, than expensive, complicated ones. Surprisingly, in many instances there is an almost inverse relationship between a product's price and its value as a beauty aid. No one wants to spend more money to look less beautiful, but this is exactly what millions of misinformed women do every day.

Most of the special beauty problems and skin disorders to be covered are usually associated with certain age groups, and they are discussed in conjunction with that age group in which they most frequently make their initial appearance. However, the age at which they first appear varies according to a number of factors, and some of them can occur at almost any age. So if you have one of these problems and it isn't covered in the chapter applicable to you, try locating it in the general index at the back of the book. In many cases, medicated products are available that will eliminate or control these special problems without the need to resort to professional help. None of the medicated products mentioned by name in this book requires a prescription. Some of these are made by large pharmaceutical companies, while others come from small specialty companies that primarily serve dermatologists. Not all of these products are kept in stock by the smaller drugstores at all times, but any one of them can be ordered for you. Don't take no for an answer if a druggist seems reluctant to order a medicated product. There are lazy druggists, just as there are lazy butchers, bakers, and candlestick-makers. In cases where you need the help of a dermatologist or a plastic surgeon, an attempt will be made to familiarize you with the options that are available to these physicians in trying to solve your special problem. A basic knowledge of both the disorder itself and the various treatments available will facilitate your dealings with these professionals, and enable them to help you more effectively.

Following this, there is an inside look at the beauty business, including its products and practitioners. This chapter will tell you frankly what is good and what is bad: what is valuable and what is useless in this field: and how this affects you personally. Finally, there is a potpourri of beauty hints, anecdotes, opinions, tips, observations, facts, and suggestions culled from notes accumulated during my twenty-five years as a practicing dermatologist.

Even though much of the beauty advice specifically applicable to you may be concentrated in one chapter, you will be better prepared for solving individual problems and anticipating future needs if you read the whole book from cover to cover. Also, if you have children or grandchildren, you will certainly want to read the chapters on childhood and adolescence. Since these young people can't or won't do this for themselves, it is your responsibility to become familiar with their beauty needs and help them look their best in the long lifetime ahead.

Before reading the chapters devoted to the practical aspects of beauty care, it is important that everyone, regardless of age or present circumstances, have a firm understanding of the fundamental principles upon which this care is based. The best place to start this search for knowledge is at the source of beauty itself, where nature provides the ultimate example of the art of being beautiful.

II A Beautiful Beginning

I was once asked by the hostess of a radio show in Chicago if standing on the head, yoga fashion, was good for the appearance. She apparently had been doing this for some time, but hadn't noticed the expected improvement. I answered her question indirectly, saying that experience had taught me the wisdom of always going along with the established principles of human physiology and, if the face would fare better down between the feet, it would have been put there in the first place.

Contrary to what the yoga devotees may think, inverting the body *decreases* circulation to the head. This is a pressure phenomenon, based on the well-known medical fact that the circulation is most sluggish through the legs and feet, the lowest parts of the body. (Ever hear of anyone having varicose veins on the upper parts of the body?) Therefore, standing on the head would slow the rate of blood flow to the face, rather than accelerate it. Standing on the head could only be of benefit in cases of circulatory insufficiency of the lower legs.

The main point of this story is that everything, including

the circulation, is arranged for maximum efficiency by the laws of nature, and can't be improved by violating natural laws. You should always respect these natural laws and try to make them work for you, rather than try to change them. In this particular instance, of course, the hostess was wasting her time.

It is amazing what the natural processes of the human body can accomplish if left to their own devices. For example, the best complexion in the world belongs to a newborn baby, and some useful lessons may be learned by seeing how nature cares for the fragile skin of a developing child. So let's begin the beauty story where it really begins—during the fetal period—and look at some of the conditions under which the skin is formed, develops, and finally becomes the perfect substance it is at birth. Here is the supreme example of nature surpassing art. You can't exactly duplicate this type of care in the postnatal period but, by following nature's example, you can come pretty close. Obviously, the closer you come to this ideal care, the better you will look at any stage of life.

First, it's very dark in the womb. If you ever thought that sunlight, any sunlight, was good for the skin, nature disagrees with you. Since sunlight is one of the skin's worst enemies, nature has wisely decreed that its development should take place in total darkness; not a single ray of light is allowed to reach the unborn child. Try to remember this the next time you are exposing your unprotected face to the sun on the beach, or by a swimming pool.

The fetal environment is also temperature-controlled, and never gets too hot or too cold. The thermostat is set at 98.6° Fahrenheit, about the same as warm water, which is also normal body temperature. Nature knows that extreme heat or cold can damage the complexion, so the temperature is always kept at this optimum level. Remember this the next time you expose yourself to freezing weather, take a facial sauna, or splash the skin with scalding water.

Nature is also a good housekeeper. The developing child's environment is kept cleaner than the operating room of any hospital, because nature knows that dirt, pollutants, chemicals, and many other noxious substances can harm the complexion. Accordingly, not one particle of foreign matter is allowed to enter nature's laboratory. As a matter of fact, this is the only time of life when the individual is completely safe from these airborne substances. Unfortunately, this situation changes abruptly when the child emerges into the dirty, polluted world its parents and grandparents have prepared for it. Remember this the next time you are out in a heavy smog or carelessly use a sanitizer or insecticide in your home.

Finally, the developing complexion never runs short of moisture, because the fetus is entirely surrounded by water; not turtle oil, honey, milk, cucumber juice, or some other exotic substance, but just plain water. Nature knows that dryness can cause problems, so this most effective precaution has been taken to assure that the skin remains moist at all times. Remember this the next time you are out on a windy day or sitting in a dry, overheated room.

These are some of the most important things that nature does to care for and perfect the complexion. However, this happy set of circumstances lasts only about thirty-eight weeks, after which the fully developed infant must leave this dermatological Garden of Eden and enter the outside world. Unless an effort is made to duplicate these prenatal conditions as closely as possible, the appearance will start to go downhill almost as soon as the baby is born, slowly and imperceptibly at first, and then more rapidly as the years go by.

As the child leaves the maternity hospital, its face is struck for the first time by direct sunlight. Simultaneously, particles of dust, dirt, and pollutants land on its exterior. If the day is windy and cold, moisture starts leaving the skin at a rapid rate: the problem is increased when the child reaches home and is deposited in an overheated nursery. It is then given a bath in water that is decidedly too hot and, as a final touch, the nursery is sprayed with a chemical disinfectant. A few days of this, of course, won't make much difference. But if this same pattern persists for a number of years, these things can affect the appearance to a remarkable extent.

Sunlight penetrates and damages the entire skin. The changes it causes are latent, which means that they don't appear right away, but only after a waiting period of many years. At first, the skin becomes somewhat coarse and leathery-looking. Later it will begin to sag and become covered with wrinkles, lines, and broken blood-vessels. If the latent damage is severe, the skin will eventually develop pigment spots, molelike growths, rough, red spots, and skin cancers. Extremes of heat and cold can cause some of these same changes, although to a lesser degree.

From the very first day of life, the skin is assaulted continually by dirt and airborne substances. This dirty film covers the skin surface and clogs the pores. After the skin matures, sweat wastes, rancid oil-gland secretions, bacteria, and stale cosmetics make their contribution. If film is allowed to build up, it can irritate the skin. The complexion then becomes blotchy and discolored, and the numbers of enlarged pores and blackheads tend to increase. The continued presence of this dirty film can also cause the skin to become dry and sensitive.

The skin deprived of moisture not only feels parched and uncomfortable but is rough to the touch and covered by fine crepey lines. In addition, it is much more susceptible to external irritants and diseases than fully moisturized skin.

Obviously, some system of regular complexion care, continued throughout life, is an absolute necessity for everyone. Otherwise, some of the unpleasant and unattractive changes just mentioned are bound to appear. Since you want to duplicate as closely as possible the advantages your skin enjoyed during the prenatal period, here are some of the things you must do to accomplish this and be as beautiful as possible.

There are two basic types of skin care, preventive and corrective. Preventive care is designed to guard the appearance against the effects of sunlight, extremes of temperatures, dirt, and airborne substances. Avoiding the hazards of heat and cold is relatively easy. These things don't just jump up at you unexpectedly; you have to seek them out and actively place yourself in jeopardy. Avoiding sunlight presents more of a problem but, even here, there are two very satisfactory solutions. You can protect yourself by staying indoors or wearing protective clothing, or you can apply a chemical sunscreen to unprotected areas. Chemical sunscreens act by selectively blocking out the wavelengths of light that damage and cause unattractive changes in the complexion.

The skin can be protected from dirt and airborne substances by applying a thin film of some material that will act as a barrier to these contaminants. Since the same substances used as moisturizers can also perform this protective function, they will be discussed in more detail in conjunction with moisturization.

The corrective measures that must be taken are only three in number. The first is proper cleansing, which means the removal of *all* foreign matter from the skin's surface and pores. The second is moisturization and protection, which means the application of some substance to the skin that will help it retain moisture and, as mentioned previously, form a barrier to protect it. The third and last is thinning, which means removal of excess dead cells from the outer portion of the skin.

Before trying any of these three basic procedures, it is essential that you thoroughly understand each one. To cleanse the skin correctly, you must remove every last bit of the dirty surface film, not just part of it. The only way you can possibly do this is with a cleanser that rinses off with water which, by definition, limits your choice to soaps and rinsable cleansers. In addition to this, your skin may require the deep cleansing effects of alcohol, which is found as an ingredient in a number of fresheners and medicated lotions. Alcohol evaporates after its cleansing job is done, so you don't have to rinse it off as you do soaps and rinsable cleansers. Soaps, rinsable cleansers, and alcohol are the heroes in the cleansing cast. The nonrinsable oils, greases, creams, and lotions that are applied to the skin and tissued off are the villains. This is because nonrinsable cleansers are very inefficient, and it is physically impossible to remove all the dirty surface film by using them. At best, they can only dilute and partially remove the contaminants covering the skin surface. If you don't believe this, try cleansing a dirty skillet with a nonrinsable cleanser and tissue. No matter how hard you cleanse, you will still have a dirty skillet. It is exactly the same with the skin surface. Something has to be used to loosen the dirt and débris, so that the entire film can be rinsed off with water. This is the only way you can get either your face or your skillet completely clean.

The principles of moisturization and protection are equally simple. All you need is a thin film of any easily applied and easily removed substance that doesn't mix with water. When this is placed on the skin, it simultaneously prevents loss of the skin's intrinsic moisture and keeps dirt and pollutants from touching the surface. The moisturizer-protectant (hereinafter called MP) products you buy in stores come in a variety of forms, such as oils, greases, lotions, and creams. In the vast majority of these, the active MP ingredient is either mineral oil or petrolatum. These are by far the most important ingredients used in formulating MP products and they are both very effective. A multitude of oils and greases from other sources are occasionally used in these products, and they, too, work very well. Consequently, it is no exaggeration to say that one of the main occupations of the cosmetic inductry is converting oils and greases into forms that look, smell, and feel better than the unadorned raw materials.

It is easy to see how oils and greases form a barrier and help protect the skin, but how can they possibly increase its moisture content? The explanation is amazingly simple. What they actually do is retard the rate of evaporation into the dry atmosphere, thereby sealing moisture into the skin. In a way, the skin moisturizes itself; these substances only create the conditions that make this possible. There is never any real shortage of supply, because water from the deeper layers is always available to the skin. A dryness problem is created only when the outer part of the skin loses moisture at too rapid a rate. It's like the spendthrift with a well-paying job who goes broke. The salary is generally adequate but, if the outgo exceeds the income for any period of time, bankruptcy results. Whether it's money or moisture, conservation is the answer in both situations. The person with money in the bank always feels better, and skin that contains the proper amount of moisture always looks better. The fully moisturized complexion is soft and smooth and shows an absence of fine crepey lines.

Thinning is the process by which the buildup of dead cells, plus their contained pigment, are removed from the skin's surface. There are two types of thinners, abrasive and chemical. The abrasive method includes the use of textured surfaces, such as washcloths, loofah sponges, brushes, and minute gritty particles, either used alone or suspended in some kind of base. Chemical thinners are used primarily to open blocked pores. There are also stronger ones that are utilized by professionals in doing deep-thinning procedures, called chemical surgery. The skin that has been properly thinned appears more translucent, and both its texture and its color are improved. In addition, the pores appear smaller and the number of blackheads is reduced. Although pore-thinning may be needed by adolescents with a tendency to enlarged pores and blackheads, overall thinning of the skin is required only by those mature women who have neglected and abused their skins during the early years.

This brief description shows how nature works its wonders on the complexion, and what you must do, in a general way, to duplicate these results. But this takes only external factors into account, and so is only part of the story. Internal factors can very definitely affect beauty. The picture wouldn't be complete without a look at how nature provides for the general health of the developing fetus. Here, too, the care is almost perfect.

Nature always provides just the right amounts of calories, vitamins, and minerals and, in addition, keeps all potentially toxic substances out of the fetal system. The weight is adjusted to the size of the body, and there are no rapid weight gains to stretch and strain the developing skin. Naturally, plenty of rest is provided, and all exercising is done in a state of weightlessness, something duplicated in later life only by scuba-diving or space-walking. If nature could dictate the ideal exercise, it would probably be swimming. Finally, nature allows the child to develop free from any physical or mental stresses. There are no problems with relatives or spouses, no financial difficulties, and no strenuous or unpleasant jobs to perform. You would also do well to emulate, to the best of your ability, the provisions nature makes for the general health during this developmental period.

Once deprived of this ideal care, the individual must begin where nature has left off. Obviously, it is impossible for anyone to exactly duplicate all these prenatal conditions but, with a little time and effort, you can obtain results that closely approximate those achieved by nature. This care should begin at birth and be continued throughout life, using the products and methods best suited to your particular age group.

With this as a theoretical background, the discussion of the practical aspects of beauty care will begin with the problems of childhood. Unfortunately, the care afforded the average child is either of poor quality or lacking altogether. The reason for this discrepancy is that a child's beauty is invariably taken for granted. This is a tragic mistake, because beauty may be totally and permanently destroyed during this critical period. On the positive side, much can be done to enhance a child's appearance and insure a beautiful future, as the following chapter will conclusively demonstrate.

III Childhood

The skin at birth anticipates, in many ways, the senile skin it will one day become. For example, both children and those in their later years have skin that is delicate and extremely dry. Thus, each individual comes full circle during the course of a lifetime. This serves to emphasize a fact that is seldom appreciated, namely, that the beauty problems of childhood can be just as serious as those at the other end of the age spectrum.

Like anything immature, the skin of the child is easily injured. It is thin and, therefore, very sensitive to temperature extremes. In addition, it lacks the protective pigment of older skin, so it is easily penetrated and damaged by sunlight. The skin of the child is also delicate, and it is easily irritated by soaps, fabrics, and the many other things with which it comes in contact during the course of an average day. The hair is fragile and very sparse during the early years. The child's pores are minute, and its sweat and oil glands are relatively inactive. The absence of oil-gland secretions, in particular, makes the child's skin extremely susceptible to the drying effects of wind and low humidity.

The skin is growing rapidly during the early years and, as it grows, it needs proper care to bring it to the full bloom of maturity.

Particular attention must be paid to protecting the skin during this period. A day on which this is neglected is an opportunity lost forever and may mean a small wrinkle or two gained somewhere down the line, at a time when the mature individual least wants or needs it. Children don't realize this, of course, but they are sowing the same seeds of destruction as adults do when they neglect routine care of the skin. Consequently, their parents or guardians must take complete responsibility during this very crucial time.

Most women have, at one time or another, looked at a friend's family photographs and found themselves fascinated by pictures of their friend as a child. Most likely, many of these showed her playing on the beach or by a swimming pool, or out in the new snow on a sparkling bright day. If you have ever had this experience, you may have consciously or unconsciously compared the child's face with that of the adult, now beginning to wrinkle and sag, and wondered how it could all happen in such a brief period of time. The answer is in the pictures. These show that, from a very early age, the child was repeatedly exposed to direct sunlight, which is by far the most damaging part of the environment. Now, the beautiful little girl in the picture is paying the terrible price for her parents' neglect.

As far as overall health and happiness are concerned, it is probably much better to allow a child to smoke or drink than to be repeatedly exposed to direct sunlight. Smoking doesn't cause wrinkles (as was once reported), and the link between smoking and lung cancer is less well substantiated than the link between sunlight and skin cancer. Alcoholic beverages have other harmful effects, of course, but wrinkles and cancer are not among them. Excessive light exposure in childhood not only ruins the appearance in later years but causes skin malignancies to boot. The body is unable to heal the damage caused by sunlight, as it sometimes does that caused by tobacco and alcohol, so this damage remains like a time-bomb in the skin, its destructive potential increasing with each additional exposure.

Children are at a disadvantage when it comes to protection from sunlight. They are not allowed to wear makeup, don't usually wear hats or gloves, and certainly won't stay under an umbrella or carry one. All these physical methods of protection are excellent for those who will use them on a regular basis, but this doesn't include children. Since youngsters are constantly out of doors, and love to be around water and snow, the total light exposure during the early years is usually substantial. It is, however, possible to obtain adequate protection with one of the chemical sunscreens. Those that come in oily or greasy bases are best for children, for two reasons. Around water, children are in and out a hundred times a day, and screens with oily or greasy bases stay on better. (It would be very difficult to reapply another kind of screen after each immersion in water.) Children are also likely to have dry skin, and sun increases this problem. The oily and greasy bases help moisturize the skin to a greater extent than the others and help prevent dryness. One sunscreen that is very suitable for children is Bain de Soleil Suntan Creme. It's not very elegant cosmetically, but children don't care about that, and it does give them excellent protection. Remember also, to apply a lip pomade containing a chemical sunscreen, and always look for the name of the active ingredient on the label before you buy one. Amyl dimethyl PABA (Para-amino-benzoic acid) is the one most frequently found in these products.

The child most susceptible to sun damage is one with light skin, heavy freckling, and reddish hair, but even black skin is susceptible to a sunburn and sun damage, although to a lesser degree. Black parents should never be deluded into thinking that the modest excess of pigment in their offspring's skins assures complete protection.

You will often hear that sunlight is good for children because it activates the Vitamin D in their skins. It is perfectly true that sunlight activates Vitamin D, but the child should get this particular vitamin from a bottle, not from a sunburn. When I was young, the vogue was to put children under a sunlamp occasionally during the winter months. This may have been done to increase the supply of Vitamin D, or possibly on the theory that the infectious microorganisms prevalent during the winter preferred pale people to tanned people. In my own case, I vividly remember taking large doses of cod-liver oil every day, so I certainly got more Vitamin D than my system could possibly use. In retrospect, those early bouts with the sunlamp certainly did me no good and by now have probably caused a few more wrinkles to appear. However, I don't blame my parents a bit. The effects of light damage were largely unknown at the time, and they were only doing what they thought was best.

Sunlight isn't the only enemy of young skin. When the skin of a young child is exposed for a prolonged period to bitterly cold weather, there is always the chance of damage due to frostbite. Dryness and chapping due to moisture-depletion, which will be discussed later in more detail, are more common occurrences during cool, windy weather. All of these things are easily preventable. They are caused in part by the fact that children are inclined to be optimists as far as weather is concerned, and they tend to brave the elements with inadequate protection. If you are the adult in charge, always insist on the wearing of earmuffs, facemasks, and heavy gloves during bitterly cold weather.

Children usually suffer no harm from environmental exposure to heat. About the only time the child's skin is subject to heat damage is when someone cleanses it using water that is too hot. Again, if you are the adult in charge of this operation, keep the water tepid, rather than hot.

There is no question about the type of product that should be used to cleanse the young skin; the answer is always soap. However, not every soap is suitable for the child's skin, with its marked tendency to sensitivity and dryness. Always use an extra-mild soap. Be sure to avoid the bars that say "Lathers in hard water" or "No bathtub ring" or "Doesn't leave a soap film." These are all detergent bars and, although they are excellent for washing your eyeglasses, they are all too harsh for the skin of the young child. Always go for the bars that don't lather quite so well in hard water, and don't worry about bathtub rings or soap films. In addition, you should never use a deodorant bar to cleanse young skin. The deodorant chemicals these bars contain can cause problems and, since the larger sweat-glands are inactive, children don't need deodorants anyway. A good part of this problem was solved recently with the demise of hexachlorophene. Likewise, heavy perfumes are sometimes a source of trouble, so avoid bar soaps containing these.

The best cleanser for infants and young children is any brand of castile soap, which is a mild soap made with pure olive oil. Try to avoid overcleansing. The slightly alkaline reaction of soap, combined with vigorous rubbing of the skin with a washcloth, will often cause increased dryness or some other untoward reaction. Cleansing time should be held to a minimum, and no washcloth should be used. The only instance in which it is permissible to use a washcloth in conjunction with soap is in the case of the older child of nine to twelve, who is beginning to show increased oil-gland activity and blackhead formation. In this situation, a washcloth can be very helpful in keeping the pores open.

The skin should always be rinsed thoroughly after cleansing to remove the last traces of soap. Older children are often careless about this, and the rinsing operation can be facilitated by taking a shower instead of a tub bath. Cleansing once, at night, is usually sufficient. However, when the child becomes older and the oil glands start to function in earnest, the face should be washed one additional time, in the morning.

There are some special aspects to the moisture problem in children. Unlike older skin, the skin of the child is easily moisturized. However, the almost total absence of natural moisturizers secreted by the oil glands means that moisture will be lost from the skin very readily under certain atmospheric conditions. So it's either feast or famine. As a consequence, children usually don't need a moisturizer during warm weather, but they need it very badly during cold weather. However, if the MP film is omitted during the summer months, the skin is left totally unprotected. Is there any risk in doing this? Probably not, because the skin of the child also seems to be less affected by airborne substances than adult skin. This is possibly due to the absence of the rancid oils and sweat wastes that are always found in abundance on mature skin. Lacking these, it is less likely that the irritant potential of the film covering the child's skin will ever reach the critical level necessary to cause problems. In a highly polluted area, however, it would be wise to take some precautions throughout the year. A thin film of almost any baby lotion applied to exposed areas will furnish adequate year-round protection.

The parts of the body covered by clothing need less moisturizing than exposed areas, but during the winter children often become dry and scaly over the entire body. If this happens, the use of soap should be cut to an absolute minimum and some type of dispersible oil added to the bath. Don't get an oil that sits on top of the water. Get one that goes into the water and forms a milky-looking mixture. Alpha Keri and Lubath are two good brands of approximately equal effectiveness.

For the moisturization and protection of exposed skin during the winter, a thin film of any baby oil will give satisfactory results. All of them are essentially mineral oil, perhaps with a little lanolin added, so the brand name isn't important. During cold weather, when there is extensive chapping of the face, the use of a heavier product is necessary. One of the best is all-purpose cold cream. Although this makes an ineffective cleanser for adults, since is it thick and nonrinsable, it is a superb moisturizer for children. It is very good for insulating the skin against extreme cold and high winds. Used indoors during the winter, it also prevents the dry air of heated rooms from extracting all of the skin's moisture.

Thinning the child's skin is unnecessary except in the special instance of pore-thinning noted previously. Although immature skin has some special quirks that must be taken into account, the skin of the child is generally easier to care for than that of any other age group. As it is with many things, including care of the complexion, life will never again be quite so simple.

Children don't use damaging chemicals on their hair and, as a consequence, are much less susceptible to hair problems than adults. Since children's hair lacks the strength of adult hair, however, it is easily pulled out by the roots or broken off by unknowing parents who are trying to care for it or style it. Young hair should not be placed under tension,

such as occurs when the hair is wrapped tightly around hair
rollers or worn as a ponytail or in braids. Various types of
clips or barrettes and rubber bands can also put tension on
the hair and pull it out. Contrary to popular opinion, vigorous combing and brushing will not make a child's hair grow;
it can only remove it, particularly if the hair is wet. In other
words, a youngster's hair will grow better and look better if
it is left entirely alone. A twice-a-week cleansing with
Johnson's Baby Shampoo is sufficient. Spray-on creme
rinses or "untanglers" are not harmful to children and help
avoid the trauma encountered in combing out little girls'
long hair. For ease of maintenance and maximum thickness,
it should be worn no longer than shoulder-length.

Children aren't generally subject to the many chronic
internal diseases that can cause such extreme changes in an
adult's appearance, but attention to their general health is
still highly important. This is particularly true of nutrition.
The infant or child is actively growing, and this means
building new tissue. Protein is the body's main building
material, and every child's diet should be high in lean meat,
poultry, fish, eggs, milk, and cheese. A minimum of fat
should be included in the diet, and just enough starches and
sugars to meet the body's energy requirements. You can't
harm a child by giving too much protein and, as any con-
tractor will tell you, it's better to have an excess of building
materials on hand than to run short halfway through the job.

Many parents either aren't able or don't know how to
provide children with the well-balanced diet they need.
Even if they do, many children are finicky eaters from
birth. For these reasons, the diet of every child should be
supplemented with a product containing the vitamins most
needed by children, namely A, C, and D. This will assure
the child's proper growth and development, especially in
those cases where there is any question of a deficiency

problem. This supplement should be continued in all instances until the growth phase is completed.

All rapid weight-gains must be avoided during childhood or else the skin's delicate tissues may be stretched and damaged. This can lead to permanent scars. It is shocking to see "stretch marks" on the thighs or abdomens of children who have been allowed to gain weight too rapidly. It is also unnecessary.

Allowing an overweight condition to persist during the developmental period is an even worse mistake. Recent evidence has shown that an obese child will form relatively more fat cells than the child of normal weight, and that these excess cells tend to be permanent. In other words, the longer the child remains overweight during the growth period, the greater the number of fat cells that will be present at maturity. Since the adult who has an increased number of fat cells removes fat from the blood and stores it at a faster rate than the adult who is not burdened with this extra tissue, fat children usually turn into fat adults. This is because the excess cells acquired during childhood make them more prone to gain weight. Because of the volume of fat, it is also much more difficult for these adults to lose weight. It's very much like the difference between emptying a bathtub one bucket at a time and trying to do the same thing with a swimming pool. This is why adults who were allowed to become overweight as children always find it very difficult to shed extra pounds or, if they do, are usually able to maintain their normal weight for only a brief period of time. They are handicapped from the beginning, and the constant effort required is just too much for them.

It's relatively easy to reduce a child's weight and keep it normal prior to the appearance of these excess fat cells. This is not the main point, however, Neither overweight children nor overweight adults are very pleasing to the eye and, in addition, the adults are much more subject to various internal diseases. This is why it is so important to keep a child's weight within normal limits during the developmental period. When you consider the consequences, allowing children to become overweight is just as bad as allowing them to overexpose themselves to the sun. In view of this, perhaps the statement made at the beginning of this chapter should be amended to read, "As far as the overall health and happiness are concerned, it is probably much better to allow a child to smoke or drink than to be repeatedly exposed to direct sunlight *or become overweight.*" It is certainly as bad as this and, as more of the harmful consequences of adult obesity become known, it may prove to be even worse. A fat child with sun-damaged skin not only has a statistically shorter lifespan but is less attractive throughout the better part of it.

This concludes the discussion of routine beauty care as it applies to children. The second section of this chapter will deal with some of the special problems encountered during childhood. This format will be retained in subsequent chapters, the first section being devoted to routine beauty care, and the second to special problems.

Of all the skin conditions prevalent during childhood, none looks worse than severe eczema. There are two types of eczema, the *seborrheic* and the *atopic.* The former is a distant relative of dandruff, and the latter is akin to the "housewife's hands" of later years. (See Chapter VI.)

Eczema is not caused by bacteria or a virus, nor is it primarily allergic in origin. Outside of a tendency to occur in families, there is no known cause. Neither type of eczema can be cured in the usual sense, but both are susceptible to some degree of control. Treatment is aimed at suppressing the symptoms and keeping the patient comfortable during the course of the disease. The duration of eczema may be months, years, or a whole lifetime. This disease will often get better and then become worse again, for no apparent reason. After continuing this irregular pattern for a variable period of time, it often disappears spontaneously.

Seborrheic eczema, also called *cradle cap* in infants, consists of a bright red eruption with sharp borders, sometimes covered with greasy-looking scales. Although the scalp is usually affected most severely, it may also appear on the face or neck, around the navel, in the groin, or between the buttocks. In rare instances, it involves almost the entire body. In cases where seborrheic eczema is confined to the scalp, a daily cleansing with a medicated shampoo may control the process. One good brand is Sebulex. For extensive eruptions on the body, Pragmatar Ointment is sometimes helpful. This is a strong medication and should never be applied full strength to a child's skin, but always diluted with water. One part of Pragmatar Ointment should be mixed with three parts of water. This can easily be done in a cup with the aid of a spoon or any other mixing instrument. A small amount of diluted ointment should be applied to all affected areas at bedtime and rinsed off the following morning.

The atopic type of eczema may appear shortly after birth. When it begins this early, the child often outgrows it by the age of two years. However, the more severe cases occur in older children. Atopic eczema characteristically affects the face, neck, and bends of the arms and legs, causing the skin of these areas to become dry and scaly. There is incessant itching, and the constant scratching frequently causes the skin to thicken. Sometimes an oral antihistamine, such as the Novahistine Elixir, is helpful in alleviating the itch. It should be used according to the manufacturer's directions.

Limiting the use of soap is one of the standard methods of treating this condition. The child is bathed only every other day. In severe cases, soap may have to be discontinued altogether. In addition, the child should wear cotton garments exclusively, and wool or synthetic fabrics should not be allowed to touch the skin. To control the inflammation and itching, a medication such as 3-percent Vioform Cream can be applied to the affected areas several times daily. This and other medications recommended for both seborrheic and atopic eczema may occasionally disagree with young patients and make the process worse instead of better. Consequently, the medications should be stopped at the first sign of irritation.

Any child with severe seborrheic or atopic eczema should be seen by a physician. Prescriptions for external and internal products containing cortisone are the basis of the medical approach to these problems. In addition, prescriptions specifically designed to control itching and other specialized forms of treatment may be prescribed. Remember, a physician can no more cure seborrheic or atopic eczema than can the parents, but medical treatment may offer a greater degree of control.

Children are the main victims of impetigo, a contagious bacterial infection. It has a predilection for the face, arms, and legs, but may occur anywhere on the body. The lesions are round to oval, with a yellowish or brownish central crust and a blistery-appearing border. The periphery of these lesions may be quite red and inflamed. The key to the treatment of impetigo lies in soaking off the crusts with warm, soapy water. In this instance, the type of soap used is immaterial. Afterwards, some type of antibiotic ointment is applied. The most effective is Neo-Polycin Ointment. The treatment should be repeated three times a day. In extensive cases, internal antibiotics administered by a physician may become necessary.

Ringworm is a fungus infection that often affects the scalp of children, where it causes bald patches. On the smooth skin, it appears as red, scaling circular lesions. When ringworm affects the skin between the toes, it is called *athlete's foot.* In this circumstance, the skin develops cracks and has a whitish appearance, and the toes may become red and swollen.

Scalp ringworm requires the care of a physician and the internal administration of a prescription antifungal drug. Ringworm of the body and athlete's foot can usually be treated successfully with Tinactin solution or cream. This medication should be applied twice daily.

Warts are caused by a virus and, since they are transmitted by physical contact, must be considered contagious. Children are more susceptible than adults, and warts are among the most difficult of childhood problems. Treatment of the child who has multiple warts is lengthy, painful, or both. Small warts can sometimes be eradicated by applying a drop of castor oil to the wart's surface and covering with adhesive tape. The treatment should be repeated nightly, and the wart kept covered with castor oil and bandaged in this fashion for four to eight weeks. Large, painful warts on the hands or feet can often be treated successfully with 40 percent salicylic acid plaster. The technique is as follows: A piece of plaster the size of the wart is cut out and the gauze backing removed. Be sure that the piece of plaster is no larger than the wart. It is then applied with the sticky side touching the wart and covered with adhesive tape to keep it in place. The plaster must be changed every twenty-four hours. After removing the old plaster, the area is cleansed with soap and water, and the dead skin scraped from the top of the wart with a penknife or scissors blade. A fresh plaster is then cut out and applied. This should be continued for two weeks, followed by a rest period of two weeks, during which no plaster is applied, and the wart is kept covered by plain adhesive tape. If the wart does not disappear after the first round of treatment, it may be repeated. Warts that prove resistant to this method must be treated by a physician. Medical treatment includes burning or cutting the wart, X-ray, and the application of strong caustics or liquid nitrogen.

Although children are born with a variety of rare birthmarks, the most common types contain blood vessels. There are two basic kinds of birthmarks: the port-wine type, which is flat and purplish in color, and the strawberry type, which is elevated and bright red. Neither of these birthmarks is susceptible to any kind of home treatment.

The port-wine type always stays about the same relative size throughout life. Various measures, such as freezing and irradiation, have been used to treat infants having these birthmarks, but none of them is very satisfactory. After the child has matured, a certain number of port-wine birthmarks may be helped by plastic surgery, but in others, there is absolutely nothing to be done, and the individual must bear the birthmark throughout life. In this case, a special makeup, such as Covermark or Erace, is very helpful.

Strawberry birthmarks will often grow very rapidly during the first few months of life, reach their maximum size, and then slowly fade away during the developmental period. The parents must learn to be patient, because it often takes quite a number of years for the blood vessels in these birthmarks to completely disappear. Occasionally one will grow very rapidly and become ulcerated. In this case, the help of a physician should be sought. All strawberry birthmarks above a certain size leave some residual scar tissue, but this can easily be removed in later years by a surgeon.

Another extremely common type of blood-vessel birthmark consists of a discrete red flare on the nape of the neck. This is harmless and never causes cosmetic problems, since it always occurs in an area covered by hair.

After childhood, potential beauty hazards increase in both number and severity, and the adult must try to anticipate these and take arms against them. This situation is further complicated by the fact that formulating methods for the adult to avoid these hazards can also be much more difficult. The main reason for this is that after the individual has physically matured, it is more difficult to use chronological age as a basis for accurate beauty guidance—adults are not as easy to categorize as children. However, this obstacle can be circumvented by means of the Personal Skin Index, which is the subject of the following chapter.

IV The Personal Skin Index

Due to its immaturity, all children's skin is very much alike, regardless of skin type. Once the skin has fully developed, however, the situation changes drastically. The skins of adults differ considerably from one another, and each needs a different kind of special care. The subject of this brief chapter is how each individual can find the specific beauty routine that is best suited to her particular skin.

The two factors responsible for the differences found in mature skins are inherited skin type and skin condition, which together determine the skin's biological age. Depending on the circumstances, this may or may not be the same as the chronological age (or age in years). Of the two, the biological age gives a much more precise indication of the skin's current status, and beauty-care recommendations made on this basis are much more accurate. For instance, you may think of yourself as a young adult in chronological terms, but you may actually have a skin that is middle-aged from a biological standpoint, or one that is still in adolescence!

For this reason, the chapters dealing with care of the mature skin have been keyed to biological rather than chronological age. Before reading these chapters, and particularly before deciding which beauty routine to follow, you should determine your skin's biological age. This will indicate the specific routine most likely to give you the best results.

To help you do this, examine the five sets of statements that follow. There are four individual statements in a set, and each statement has opposite it a numerical value ranging from 1 to 4. Pick the one statement in each of the five sets that comes closest to describing the present condition of your skin, and note its numerical value. Add these five figures and the result will be your own Personal Skin Index, or PSI, which is simply your skin's biological age expressed as a numerical value. After this, turn to the summaries of skin-care routines at the end of this chapter. Here you will find a range of PSI values and a summary of each of the adult beauty routines. The one containing your PSI is the one you should use. The purpose of the summary is to familiarize you in advance with the framework of your routine, and the summaries of routines used by other biological age groups will be helpful in anticipating any future adjustments.

As an actual example of how the PSI is used, if your PSI is 12, you should use the routine recommended for young adults. If it is 13, you should use the one recommended for middle age.

1. *Oil Glands and Pores*

    A. Oily skin, large pores, with or without   1
            tendency to blackheads and blemishes

    B. Mixed oily-dry, pores medium or enlarged   2
            only in certain areas

    C.   Normal with medium pores, tendency to   3
           dryness during cool weather

    D.   Dry or very dry skin, tendency to enlarged   4
           pores, occasional blackheads and
           whiteheads

2. *Pigment and Blood Vessels*

    A.   Dark or medium skin, with even color   1

    B.   Light skin with tendency to freckles   2

    C.   Color uneven, face and/or neck with a few   3
           enlarged blood vessels

    D.   "Liver spots" on hands or face, many   4
           enlarged or "broken" blood vessels

3. *Resistance*

    A.   Never any problems using makeup or skin   1
           care products

    B.   Skin sensitive at certain times, cannot use   2
           some products

    C.   Skin moderately sensitive, easily irritated by   3
           a number of products

    D.   Skin extremely sensitive and irritable,   4
           tolerates only a few carefully selected
           products

4. *Skin Texture*

    A. Skin uniformly soft and smooth   1

    B. Smooth with occasional patchy roughness   2

    C. Somewhat coarse and rough   3

    D. Leathery with localized rough, red spots   4

5. *Skin Contour*

    A. No lines or wrinkles   1

    B. Few small lines about eyes and/or
            forehead   2

    C. Shallow wrinkles, with or without moderate   3
            sagging

    D. Deep wrinkles, extensive sagging   4

SUMMARY OF DAILY SKIN CARE ROUTINES BY BIOLOGICAL AGE GROUP

PSI 5 – 7
CHAPTER V — ADOLESCENCE

	A.M.	P.M.
M	Soap Alcoholic freshener Moisturizer-protectant	Soap Medicated lotion
T	Soap Alcoholic freshener Moisturizer-protectant	Soap Medicated lotion
W	Soap Alcoholic freshener Moisturizer-protectant	Soap Medicated lotion
TH	Soap Alcoholic freshener Moisturizer-protectant	Soap Medicated lotion
F	Soap Alcoholic freshener Moisturizer-protectant	Soap Medicated lotion
S	Soap Alcoholic freshener Moisturizer-protectant	Soap Medicated lotion
S	Soap Alcoholic freshener Moisturizer-protectant	Soap Medicated lotion

SUMMARY OF DAILY SKIN CARE ROUTINES BY BIOLOGICAL AGE GROUP

PSI 8 – 12
CHAPTER VI — YOUNG ADULTHOOD

	A.M.	P.M.
M	Soap Alcoholic freshener Moisturizer-protectant	Soap Alcoholic freshener Moisturizer-protectant
T	Soap Alcoholic freshener Moisturizer-protectant	Soap Alcoholic freshener Moisturizer-protectant
W	Soap Alcoholic freshener Moisturizer-protectant	Soap Alcoholic freshener Moisturizer-protectant
TH	Soap Alcoholic freshener Moisturizer-protectant	Soap Alcoholic freshener Moisturizer-protectant
F	Soap Alcoholic freshener Moisturizer-protectant	Soap Alcoholic freshener Moisturizer-protectant
S	Soap Alcoholic freshener Moisturizer-protectant	Soap Alcoholic freshener Moisturizer-protectant
S	Soap Alcoholic freshener Moisturizer-protectant	Soap Alcoholic freshener Moisturizer-protectant

SUMMARY OF DAILY SKIN CARE ROUTINES BY BIOLOGICAL AGE GROUP

PSI 13 – 17
CHAPTER VII — MIDDLE AGE

	A.M.	P.M.
M	Moisturizer-protectant	Soap Alcoholic freshener Moisturizer-protectant
T	Moisturizer-protectant	Soap Thinner Moisturizer-protectant
W	Moisturizer-protectant	Soap Alcoholic freshener Moisturizer-protectant
TH	Moisturizer-protectant	Soap Alcoholic freshener Moisturizer-protectant
F	Moisturizer-protectant	Soap Thinner Moisturizer-protectant
S	Moisturizer-protectant	Soap Alcoholic freshener Moisturizer-protectant
S	Moisturizer-protectant	Soap Alcoholic freshener Moisturizer-protectant

SUMMARY OF DAILY SKIN CARE ROUTINES BY BIOLOGICAL AGE GROUP

PSI 18 – 20
CHAPTER VIII — THE LATER YEARS

	A.M.	P.M.
M	Moisturizer-protectant	Rinsable cleanser Moisturizer-protectant
T	Moisturizer-protectant	Rinsable cleanser Thinner Moisturizer-protectant
W	Moisturizer-protectant	Rinsable cleanser Moisturizer-protectant
TH	Moisturizer-protectant	Rinsable cleanser Moisturizer-protectant
F	Moisturizer-protectant	Rinsable cleanser Thinner Moisturizer-protectant
S	Moisturizer-protectant	Rinsable cleanser Moisturizer-protectant
S	Moisturizer-protectant	Rinsable cleanser Moisturizer-protectant

V Adolescence
(PSI 5-7)

The adolescent skin is a flawed masterpiece. On the positive side, it is rapidly maturing and is approaching a peak as far as strength, resiliency, and overall resistance are concerned. Even if the skin has been neglected and abused during childhood, the visible effects of skin damage are yet to make their appearance, The skin is taut and free from sagging, and there are no lines, wrinkles, or broken blood-vessels. The texture is excellent and the color is even. The oil glands reach their maximum output during this period, and the skin is easily moisturized. In contrast to the child's dry skin, the skin of the adolescent is soft and smooth. In many ways, it will never look this good again.

On the negative side, the increased oiliness makes the face shine like a headlight, and both the skin and hair have a vaguely unclean look about them. This impression has a basis in fact, because oily skin and hair attract and hold more dirt. The pores of the adolescent skin are enlarged, and there is a marked increase in the number of blackheads and whiteheads.

Adolescence is a unique period of life as far as the appearance is concerned. With the onset of puberty, there is a radical shift in the hormone balance, and suddenly all sorts of things begin to happen in rapid succession. The most important changes, as far as beauty is concerned, are the effects of this hormonal shift on the oil glands and pores. The oil glands enlarge to several times their normal size and begin pouring out copious amounts of oil. The necks of the pores thicken, and the partial obstruction that follows causes them to enlarge. The combination of increased oil-flow and pore-blockage causes the blackheads and whiteheads so characteristic of this age. These problems are fairly constant in boys, but in girls, they sometimes seem to wax and wane with the menstrual cycle.

This same hormonal change also causes the large sweat-glands to become active for the first time, and hair begins to appear in places where it never grew before. This is the age when the skin is first introduced to shaving aids, deodorants, makeup, and other products with which it will have to contend throughout life.

In addition to these bodily changes, the lifestyle of the adolescent is in a state of flux, and behavior patterns change as the child struggles toward adulthood. The habits formed during this period will persist in many instances for the rest of the individual's life. Even though it is a time of twilight for parental authority, those adults with whom the teenager has contact can still exert a tremendous influence for good or bad. This is an important responsibility, because the habits that crystallize during adolescence can affect the health, appearance, and happiness for many years to come.

Teenagers always seem to go to extremes, and the way in which they handle environmental exposure is a case in point. If they are not secreted in their rooms with the radio blaring, they are out exposing their unprotected bodies to the sun, sometimes to a degree approaching totality. On any warm summer day, you will see hordes of adolescents, clothed in the merest nothing, frantically trying to acquire a tan. As in childhood, even a bad sunburn has very little visible aftermath. Yet, although the damage remains latent during the adolescent period, it is still there, and the piper must be paid sooner or later. Really severe sunburn, with acute redness and blistering, seems to be particularly common among teenagers. I think this is due to the fact that so many of them believe that covering their bodies and faces with such things as baby oil, cocoa butter, coconut oil, etc., will keep them from burning and increase tanning. Both of these assumptions are entirely false. None of these substances affords any sun protection at all; neither do they affect the rate of tanning. The advertisements that read, "Tan fast with So-and-so," which are usually for substances like those just mentioned, tend to reinforce this mistaken impression.

One reason there are so many adolescent sun-buffs is that sunlight does help alleviate some of the skin problems prevalent at this age. Sun exposure helps decrease oiliness, and the peeling and thinning that accompany a mild sunburn free a number of blackheads and help reduce pore size. These benefits last only a short while, so the exposure must be repeated at regular intervals to prevent a relapse. In the winter, these same teenagers will often resort to a sunlamp. Regardless of whether the light is natural or artificial, teenagers who indulge in this sort of thing are trading a superficial and temporary improvement for damage that is deep and permanent. Many adolescents are not aware that their complexions can be helped to an equal or even greater extent by other measures, such as cleansers and medicated products, which are perfectly safe.

Since teenagers expose themselves to the sun more than any other group, and usually eschew any form of physical protection, such as hats and gloves, an effective chemical sunscreen should be made available to them at all times. The most suitable screens for this age group are those containing PABA. Practically all of these contain alcohol and are, therefore, somewhat drying, but this is usually more of an asset than a liability at this age. Representative brand names of PABA-containing products are PreSun and Ultrabloc. The only drawback to these highly effective sunscreens is their tendency to stain clothing but, with careful application, this is not too difficult to avoid. The screen should be applied liberally to all exposed areas, including the hands and neck.

The teenager who is adequately protected won't get much of a tan, and this often leads to disappointment. However, by using one of the "quick tans," "bronzers," or "indoor tans," a simulated tan may be acquired in a matter of hours. These products contain substances that only stain the skin, so they are completely safe. Most of them have, in addition, some type of chemical sunscreen.

Teenagers characteristically show a similar disregard for other environmental hazards. They are often out and about, usually without adequate protection, on bitterly cold days, when more prudent adults stay indoors. They are also the group most likely to abuse their skins with facial saunas, hot towels, and other forms of extreme heat. Much of this misuse of heat can be attributed to the erroneous theory that heat opens the pores and makes blackheads easier to remove. The truth is that heat doesn't open the pores to any extent, and that water actually does most of the work when it comes to softening blackheads and facilitating their removal. In this case, lukewarm or tepid water will work just as well as hot water, and it is infinitely easier on the skin. For greater softening effect and easier removal, the wetting time should be increased, not the temperature.

Since the adolescent skin attracts dirt so readily, proper cleansing is very important. As there is absolutely no way to permanently stem the flow of oil, the solution to the oiliness problem lies in the use of stronger cleansers and more frequent cleansing. The products needed to handle adolescent cleansing problems include detergent soaps, alcoholic fresheners, and medicated lotions.

This is the only time of life full-strength detergent cleansers can safely be used on the skin. All affected areas, including the back and chest, should be cleansed with a detergent soap twice a day—no more and no less. Over-cleansing with detergents can lead to skin irritation, and this often makes things worse instead of better. The choice of detergent bars is limited; it is difficult to find one that does not contain a deodorant chemical, or that is not superfatted with some "cream" ingredient. Deodorant chemicals are of absolutely no benefit to the adolescent complexion, and they can sometimes cause allergies. Superfatting ingredients are undesirable because these additives all reduce cleansing power. Soaps and other cleansers containing a variety of medications are vigorously promoted to teenagers, but medication incorporated into a soap, whether in bar or in paste form, can't possibly stay on the skin long enough to do it any good—it's rinsed away! Consequently, all medicated cleansers are a complete waste of money. One detergent bar soap that seems to do a good job is Vel. Moreover, it doesn't contain any deodorant chemicals, superfatting ingredients, or medications. If the skin becomes too dry during the winter, a switch may be made temporarily to one of the detergent-based rinsable lotions, such as Phisoderm or Hyperphase. The skin should be rinsed well after using any detergent-based cleanser, either in a shower or with several changes of fresh water. In cases where blackheads are particularly numerous, an ordinary washcloth may be used in conjunction with the cleanser to help clear obstructed pores.

A freshener containing alcohol is indispensable in caring for the adolescent complexion. (You can make a very acceptable one by mixing one part rubbing alcohol to four parts water.) Alcohol is very effective in removing the last traces of oil and dirt from the pores. If the freshener is simply patted on, this action is lost, so the skin must be wiped with a saturated pad. This may be done once or twice daily, as required, to control oiliness. All adolescents should use an alcoholic freshener in the morning after cleansing with soap. A small minority of teenagers is free from the usual problems of extreme oiliness and blackheads. In these special instances, an alcoholic freshener may also be used after the bedtime cleansing with soap. However, those with typical adolescent skin should use a medicated lotion instead of a freshener at bedtime.

Medicated lotions, which may be either liquids or semisolid gels, are similar to alcoholic fresheners, but differ in that they all contain a chemical pore-thinner. Medicated lotions are extremely helpful in controlling oiliness and the large numbers of small blackheads that plague the adolescent skin.

To use a medicated lotion, wipe the skin clean with a saturated cotton pad. Then saturate a fresh pad and simply pat it on the affected areas. This leaves a slight excess of chemical thinner on the skin after the alcohol evaporates. This excess should be allowed to remain on the skin overnight and washed off with soap the next morning. It is better to use these medicated products at bedtime, rather than in the morning, because they should not be used under MP films or makeup. It is also better if they are used only once a day, instead of twice a day, as suggested by many manufacturers. This way, the skin is allowed some time each day to rest and recuperate. With this regime, MP films and makeup can be freely used during the day. If this limited once-a-day usage does not result in improvement, it usually means that an early acne is present, and other appropriate measures are then indicated. Bonne Bell Ten-0-Six is a medicated lotion that seems to give good results. Other products of this type include presaturated pads packaged in tins or jars, but these are all much less economical than the plain lotions.

When large isolated blackheads prove resistant to routine care, teenagers sometimes become frantic and start digging and squeezing the skin with their nails. This should be avoided, because it can cause permanent pore-enlargement. If a large blackhead in a particularly prominent place must be removed, do it with a blackhead-extractor, not with the fingers. These instruments are available at many drugstores and all surgical supply stores. Before using the extractor, the area should be moistened by the application of a wet cotton pad for four or five minutes. Then the blackhead should be centered in the opening of the extractor and firm pressure applied. Whiteheads should be left entirely alone. Never try to open them with pins or other makeshift instruments. They will in time go away by themselves. Another common mistake made by teenagers is the reliance on cosmetic masques for cleansing and pore-thinning. (See Chapter VIII.) These products have only marginal effectiveness along these lines and therefore are of little use to the adolescent.

Teenagers don't ordinarily require extra moisturization and protection, because their skins usually produce more than enough oil to handle these things without outside help. However, since the skin requires extra cleansing at this age, it sometimes becomes very dry during cool weather. If this happens, an MP film can help correct the situation and also insulate and protect the skin during periods of extreme cold. A thin film of any light mineral oil or baby oil will do the job adequately. It should always be applied after cleansing in the morning. The typical adolescent skin usually doesn't require any kind of MP film at bedtime or during the warm months.

A light liquid makeup won't aggravate complexion problems, particularly if it is of the water-based, oil-free variety. However, some kind of MP film should always be applied first. Adolescents should never, under any circumstances, use heavy, greasy makeup, even though it admittedly does a better job of hiding complexion problems. It requires more cleansing to remove, and this may trigger an adverse reaction in a skin that is already being cleansed and manipulated to the limit. Some teenagers go to the other extreme and are afraid to use makeup or MP films for fear they will "clog" the pores. This apprehension is groundless. Pores are filled not with air but with varying amounts of things that are much less desirable and more difficult to remove than either makeup or MP films. Removing the débris that fills the adolescent pores and replacing it with something cleaner never harmed any skin.

Hair is very special to most teenagers. Many young girls are almost compulsive in their urge to constantly do something to it. Any bathroom used by an adolescent female (males, too, nowadays!) tends to be crammed with bottles of all sizes and shapes, containing shampoos, conditioners, and so forth. These are all innocuous enough, but there are many things teenagers do to their hair that are definitely harmful. Some spend a good part of the day with their hair wound tightly around rollers, and the tension this causes can pull hair out by the roots. The rest of the day is often spent manipulating or abusing the hair in some other manner. It is weakened by the excessive use of hot-air dryers and hot curlers, and then broken off in quantity by combing, brushing, ratting, or other styling procedures. All of the hair lost in these ways can be saved simply by holding tension, heat, and mechanical trauma to an absolute minimum.

Teenagers are subject to few really serious hair problems, but one that is confined almost exclusively to the adolescent period is that which occurs following the ingestion of large amounts of Vitamin A. Many teenagers have heard that this will help solve complexion problems, so they often treat themselves with amounts that are far in excess of their daily requirements. This doesn't help the complexion to any extent, but it can cause a severe hair-loss problem. A teenager should never take more than the recommended daily dose of any vitamin.

Parents often ask if long hair that touches the forehead or upper back can make skin problems worse in these areas. The answer is that it doesn't, provided the hair is kept scrupulously clean. Short hair is always preferable to long hair because it is much easier to keep clean, but otherwise there is no definite correlation between hair length and the number of blemishes. To maintain the proper degree of cleanliness, it may be necessary for a teenager whose scalp and hair are very oily to shampoo daily. This frequency is never harmful to the hair, as long as a mild, nonmedicated shampoo is used. Johnson's Baby Shampoo is very suitable, and is particularly valuable to teenagers with fine hair.

Even if the hair is thick and healthy, and the complexion flawless, there are two beauty disabilities peculiar to this age that may throw the teenager into an emotional decline. This is caused by the advent, sometimes simultaneously, of visual and dental problems that necessitate the wearing of glasses and braces.

Although eyeglass frames are much more attractive and stylish than they once were, contact lenses are preferred by most teenagers. The new, soft contact lenses are especially popular and can be worn by almost anyone, with the exception of those having a high degree of astigmatism. The main advantages over the older, hard lenses are greater ease of wearing and more beautiful, natural-looking eyes. Both of these advantages are based on the single most important characteristic of soft lenses: the fact that they are less irritating to the eyes than hard lenses. These new lenses can be worn comfortably almost from the first day, and are more suitable for intermittent wearing or alternation with glasses. They can also be worn for longer periods of time without causing discomfort or redness. Most important, the eyes and face of the wearer are not distorted by an unattractive squint, something that occurs all too frequently with hard lenses. The major disadvantage of soft lenses seems to be the required use of a cumbersome cleaning apparatus.

Although braces have become somewhat less massive in recent years, and hence less conspicuous, there is still nothing in the field of orthodontics with an invisibility comparable to contact lenses. Braces are still unsightly and a definite social handicap to the self-conscious teenager. However, use of removable braces is becoming more common, and some of these appliances are now made of plastic instead of the highly obtrusive metal. Still, the average teenager who needs braces must resign herself to a mouth full of metallic bands and wires. Orthodontists seem to agree that allowing the metal to become dirty and dull usually detracts from the overall appearance more than the braces themselves. Cleansing the braces twice a day, after breakfast and supper, with a soft toothbrush, is usually adequate. The braces and spaces between the teeth should be thoroughly syringed at bedtime with a Water Pik. This régime will not only keep the wires and bands clean and bright but promote healthy gums.

Teenagers are generally a healthy lot. This is fortunate, because most of them have very little concern for regular medical checkups, and they are all prone to ignore advice on the subject of health, whether it comes from the parents or a physician. However, there are some special health needs at this time that should not be ignored. Diet is one of the problem areas. The adolescent, like the child, needs large amounts of protein building-material. Teenagers should concentrate on lean meat, poultry, and eggs, but avoid fish, milk, and cheese, because these classes of foods sometimes seem to worsen complexion problems. The high-carbohydrate foods also do this, so their use should be curtailed during this period. The starchy carbohydrate foods don't seem to be as bad as those containing sugar. Candies, soft drinks, and desserts should be severely limited, particularly those containing chocolate. However, dietetic or sugarfree substitutes are available in many of these categories, and are usually well-tolerated. Also, salt that doesn't contain iodine should be used in place of the iodized type. (Iodine is one of the minerals that can make blemishes or an acne problem more severe. See Chapter VI, p. 74.)

Incidentally, the old idea that fried and fatty foods are bad for the complexion has absolutely no basis in fact. Despite evidence to the contrary, the myth that these foods increase oil-gland activity is still with us. Anyone who doesn't believe this *is* a myth should try taking a couple of tablespoons of vegetable oil internally at bedtime; they won't find their skin any oilier the following morning.

Since adolescents are notorious for their irregular and sometimes bizarre eating habits, a multiple-vitamin preparation should always be taken daily to guard against the borderline deficiencies so frequent at this age. Be sure to buy a product that doesn't contain trace minerals, as these can definitely aggravate complexion problems. The mineral most likely to do this is iron. Vitamin supplements containing high concentrations of iron, in both liquid and tablet form, are sold in response to advertisements proclaiming that "women need more iron than men do." However, a well-balanced diet always furnishes enough iron to meet any female need. A teenager should never take iron in any form unless it is specifically prescribed by a physician for iron-deficiency anemia.

Teenagers should grow up, certainly, but not out. The combination of rapid growth and weight gain makes the body expand in all directions, and this is apt to cause skin damage and stretch marks. This is also the teenager's last chance to minimize the number of fat cells she will carry for the rest of her life. The eating habits during the early part of this period make the final determination as to whether it will be difficult or easy to shed those extra pounds in later years when the body has such a strong affinity for them.

Other health problems stem from the adolescent tendency to be immoderate in all things, and this is particularly true of rest and exercise. The teenager may get very little sleep at all, or may hibernate like a bear for days on end. The amount of regular exercise may be virtually nil, or it may be overdone to the point where it causes physical exhaustion. Regular and sensible habits of both sleep and exercise at this age are essential. Irregularity in either can affect not only the general health and development but also the complexion.

Parents who are keen observers frequently cite irregular sleep and "trying to do too much" as being the two most important factors in determining whether their teenager's complexion is clear or covered with blemishes. There is little doubt that a regular schedule is just as important as good skin care in keeping a blemish problem under control.

Of all the special problems encountered during adolescence, acne is by far the most important in terms of its effects on the appearance.

To what stage does a complexion problem have to progress before it can be called acne? Most dermatologists would agree that an acne condition is present when the small red blemishes surrounding the blocked pores become tender, swollen, and filled with infected material.

The trouble starts the moment the excess oil and thickened pore neck conspire to form a blackhead. This partially blocks the pore, and results in a low-grade bacterial infection within the oil gland. The flow of oil is like a river, and pollution and bacterial proliferation are much more likely when the current is slowed. Once the pore is completely blocked, this chronic infection within the oil gland quickly becomes acute. If the infection is allowed to proceed, it will break out of the oil gland and destroy some of the surrounding tissue. This is what causes the pits and scars that are so often associated with uncontrolled acne. The first goal of acne treatment is to widen the pore neck, remove the obstructing blackhead, and restore normal oil-flow. The second is to combat the infection. It must be borne in mind that acne is not curable in the sense that the cause can be eliminated. So the teenager must be satisfied with controlling the process and trying to prevent scarring. Consequently, any of the measures used to combat acne must be continued until the disease has completely disappeared.

The individual treatment of acne is, in many ways, a continuation and extension of the measures used to handle adolescent complexion problems. Detergent soaps, alcoholic fresheners, and medicated lotions are also the basic tools used in controlling acne. Likewise, proper diet, sensible rest and exercise, and freedom from mental stress are important to the acne victim. It was once believed that adolescent acne bore some relation to the degree of sexual activity. There is not a grain of truth in this; the disease affects both the saint and the swinger with equal severity.

If the adolescent skin does develop acne, the only change of any consequence that need be made in the routine is the introduction of abrasive cleansers and stronger medicated products. An abrasive cleanser should replace the detergent bar at bedtime. Brasivol is a good product of this type. It comes in three grades: fine, medium, and rough. The fine and medium grades are easier on the skin and generally give the best results. Another advantage of this product is that it doesn't contain any of the superfluous medications found in many abrasive cleansers. The skin should be rinsed thoroughly after using the cleanser. (The bedtime alcoholic freshener is omitted if the teenager is using one of these abrasive products.)

After drying the skin, one of the medicated products made specifically for acne should be applied and left on overnight. These products differ in several respects from the medicated lotions. First, and most important, they are never used on a pad for cleansing, because they usually contain far less alcohol, or none at all. Another significant difference is that the chemical thinners found in these products are much stronger than those found in medicated lotions. Komed, which is also sold under the name Microsyn, is one that seems to work well in early acne. For more advanced acne, Transact, a medicated gel, gives good results. The last traces of these products should be removed in the morning with a detergent bar soap, rather than an abrasive cleanser, since using an abrasive product more than once a day sometimes causes the skin to become irritated.

After rinsing and using an alcoholic freshener in the usual way, the skin is allowed to recuperate for the remainder of the day before its bedtime treatment. However, if the skin becomes dry during cold weather, it is not only permissible, but actually beneficial, to wear some kind of MP film during the day. In addition, a colored foundation or other light makeup may be used. There are a number of dual-purpose products containing both medication and makeup, such as Fostril and Clearasil, for those who wish to use a medicated product during the day. This schedule is more convenient in some instances, and there is no objection to this practice as long as one of these products is not used again at bedtime. As a rule, twenty-four hours of continuous medication is too much for any skin.

It is particularly important that acne lesions containing infected material not be picked or squeezed. This can force the material deeper into the skin and increase the pitting and scarring. Parents should make every effort to keep their teenagers from doing this but, if these efforts fail, it is usually a good idea to seek professional help.

Controlling the infection with internally administered antibiotics represents the most important medical contribution to the treatment of acne. Relatively small doses of antibiotic can cause an almost immediate improvement, but the acne victim must usually be kept on a maintenance dose until the acute phase of the condition subsides. This may be only a few months in some cases, but in others it is a matter of years. However, side effects are few if the patient is carefully supervised, and this treatment procedure is generally recognized as safe.

For older girls, certain brands of birth-control pills are sometimes prescribed, and these can be most effective in controlling a severe acne. Birth control pills are *never* given to normally developing girls under 16 because they can stunt the growth. (They are used sometimes to retard the rate of growth in cases where it is too rapid and there is danger of becoming abnormally tall.) All birth control pills are mixtures of different types of estrogens and progesterone in varying ratios. There are not only these qualitative differences, but they differ quantitatively in the absolute amounts of these individual components. (See Chapter VI, page 81.)

Dermatologists and other physicians can also do various minor surgical procedures, such as removing blackheads and small cysts, and opening or treating in various ways the pustular lesions that appear in severe acne. In addition, many give treatments designed to peel the skin and open the pores, such as the application of dry-ice slush. Although many dermatologists still use X-ray and ultraviolet light in the treatment of acne, it is better to avoid such procedures. Either of these may improve the acne temporarily, but both can cause latent skin damage, just as natural sunlight does. In the opinion of many, the advent of antibiotics and the other forms of acne treatment now available make the use of any skin irradiations antiquated and unnecessary.

Although improvement under medical care is usually considerable, a physician cannot cure acne any more than the patient can cure it at home. Treatment is considered successful if the process is controlled and most of the scarring and pitting prevented. Having acne during adolescence is bad enough, but having to bear the permanent disfigurement it can cause is many times worse.

Tinea versicolor is a type of fungus infection that occurs frequently in adolescence. It appears as round, slightly scaly spots, with a white or tan color. It is seen most often on the back, chest, and upper arms, and it spreads slowly to adjoining areas, so that after several years a good portion of the body may be involved. The teenager's main complaint is usually that the skin pigment is being "eaten away." They most often seek treatment during the summer, after having been denied admission to the local swimming pool because of their very noticeable skin problem.

A saturated solution of sodium hyposulfite, which can be compounded by any pharmacist, will usually eradicate this infection. It should be applied daily after the bath, and treatment should be continued for at least a month. Even if this gets rid of the fungus, it will often be several months before the pigment returns. This disease is often confused with a permanent loss of pigment called vitiligo.

The change in hormone balance at puberty causes existing moles to grow and new moles to appear. The majority of these may be disregarded, and it is not necessary to remove them unless they become irritated by clothing or are constantly being struck by combs and brushes. About the only type of mole that should be checked by a physician is the so-called *junction nevus*. This mole is flat, rather than elevated, pitch black in color, and rarely contains hairs. Although a mole corresponding to this description may be present from birth, it will rarely grow or show malignant changes prior to puberty. The malignant form of this mole is called a melanoma, and it is extremely dangerous. If an adolescent has a junction nevus or develops one at puberty, a professional opinion should be sought immediately. In most cases, only periodic observation is required. If one of these moles shows any suspicious changes, however, wide surgical excision is invariably recommended.

Most teenagers are fond of the wide-open spaces and growing things, but this fondness is not always reciprocal, so they are frequent victims of poison ivy. This always breaks out in an irregular, patchy fashion; the skin may become red and swollen, or there may be streaks of blisters on any part of the body. This pattern is sometimes confusing, even to the specialist. In severe cases, the eyes may become so swollen they are almost closed, or there may be only one or two large blisters on the fingers.

There is no reliable preventive for poison ivy, so once it appears, it is too late to do anything but ride it out as comfortably as possible. The extent of the eruption is always determined at the time of contact; you cannot spread it by scratching, even if you break one of the blisters and touch its contained fluid.

The first rule of treating poison ivy is to avoid making the inflammation any worse by applying home remedies that are too strong. Most of the cases that find their way to the doctor's office are suffering more from the effects of indiscriminate medication than from the effects of poison ivy. Milk, chilled in the refrigerator, makes a soothing cold compress, and can be used as often as necessary to stop itching. In the interim between compresses, plain calamine lotion may be applied to the affected areas. In really severe cases, internal and external medications prescribed by a physician can shorten the course of this plant allergy by a considerable margin. The medical profession continues to work on ways to protect the many people who are sensitive to this plant, but it has yet to come up with a practical solution. It doesn't sound very erudite, but staying on the sidewalk is the best advice dermatologists have to offer at this time.

Dandruff is related to the seborrheic eczema found in children. Although it looks unattractive, it doesn't affect the hair and won't cause hair loss. However, those with severe dandruff often scratch the scalp, and this can break off large numbers of hairs. It may also cause a scalp infection, which is often more difficult to control than the dandruff. This disease is another of the large group of skin afflictions that physicians can't cure in a permanent sense but can only control. The best dandruff shampoos available are Head and Shoulders, Selsun Blue, and Ionil T. These should be used three times a week at first but, after the dandruff is under control, once or twice weekly is usually sufficient. If shampoos alone don't control the dandruff, a physician's help becomes necessary. The products prescribed for dandruff usually contain cortisone and are rather inconvenient to use, because they must be applied to the scalp and left overnight. The shampoo route is definitely the lesser nuisance, especially if the hair is worn in one of the more intricate styles.

Regardless of whether it is a shampoo or a prescription given by a physician, all dandruff remedies tend to lose their effectiveness over a period of time. Consequently, if the dandruff persists, it is usually necessary to change remedies every so often. Many of those who have dandruff feel that either physical exhaustion or mental stress can definitely aggravate it. Others blame hair spray or some other hair product, but these generally have no effect on dandruff, for better or worse. Although dandruff frequently accompanies acne, there is no direct relationship, and the flakes that fall either on the face or back don't cause or aggravate acne, as some seem to think.

The end of adolescence usually finds the emerging young adult full of high hopes for the future. However, this boundless optimism should be tempered with a degree of caution, for both the best and worst are yet to come.

VI Young Adulthood
(PSI 8-12)

The condition of the skin, like athletic prowess, usually reaches its peak during young adulthood. It's true that we often see older women whose skin is beautiful, and older athletes who still perform magnificently, but these are the exceptions. If a certain level of conditioning were required for beauty, as it is for participation in competitive athletics, many women would be retired to the sidelines at a very early age.

A young adult who expects to stay active in the beauty game would be wise to devote a little extra time to the appearance. According to nature's biological clock, after adolescence the skin has already passed its peak and is starting to decline. If early warning signs are ignored, the descent will be very rapid. With appropriate care, however, deterioration may be slowed almost to a standstill, and beauty kept intact for many years.

Many different skin types are found within the bounds of this age group. Some young adults still have large pores and skin that is oilier than that of the oiliest adolescent. In others, the dryness of middle age is already present. To further confuse matters, certain areas of an individual's skin may seem dry, while others seem oily. Although the skin at the beginning of young adulthood is usually in excellent condition, things may change considerably before the end of this period.

The major difference between adolescents and young adults as far as skin is concerned, is that the older group shows less oiliness and has smaller pores. One of the beauty advantages young adults have is that at this age the rate of oil secretion is neither too fast nor too slow, but just right. There is also less tendency to thickening of the pore necks, and the average young adult has few, if any, blackheads. On the other hand, the skin of the young adult may not be the flawless article it was only a few years before. It is not as soft and smooth as that of the adolescent, and there is usually some dryness, especially during cool weather. The color of the complexion may appear slightly uneven due to an increase in pigment. The skin may also be somewhat more sensitive and irritable at this age, especially after exposure to the sun, wind, or extreme cold. Under these circumstances, a favorite skin-care or makeup product may not feel as comfortable as it once did.

As far as more profound skin changes are concerned, the young adult is in good shape in some areas, and not so good in others. The skin is still strong, taut, and resilient. There is hardly any sagging, and the fat pads underlying the skin are still of adequate thickness. This is fortunate, because these fat pads will help delay the appearances of wrinkling for a few more years at least, even though some degree of skin damage is inevitably already present. But superficial wrinkles may be even now starting to appear, particularly in areas where the pull of the facial muscles has caused the greatest strain on the skin. Young adults first notice these wrinkles around the eyes and mouth and in the center of the forehead, which are the areas most frequently used in making facial expressions. These tiny creases are almost insignificant in the beginning but, for most women, they are a chilling portent of things to come. In some young adults, there is already a shift in the color of the complexion toward the red end of the spectrum, due to a slight dilation of the skin's blood vessels. Toward the end of young adulthood, the complexion may even take on a ruddy look. These changes all give fair warning that the thrust of beauty maintained so effortlessly during adolescence is now beginning to lose its momentum, and definitely needs a push.

During young adulthood, the ovarian function begins the gradual decline that will culminate some years hence in menopause. Along with this, the body has more of a tendency to attract and hold fat, and this makes it difficult to keep the figure in shape. Even the eating habits of young adults differ from those of adolescents, and there is the ever-present possibility of abnormal weight changes and other problems related to the nutritional status. A career, marriage, homemaking, and children may all enter the picture at this age, and under their influence, the life-pattern undergoes a tremendous change. New habits of rest and exercise appear in response to new situations, as do new problems and their attendant stresses and tensions. All of these can affect beauty in a number of ways. It is paradoxical that at this time, when the appearance is beginning to need a little more attention, the average young adult simply has too many other things to worry about and too many other things to do.

On the average, young adults are probably exposed to fewer environmental hazards than adolescents. They tend to make up for it, however, by throwing caution to the winds on weekends and vacations, and severe cases of sunburn are very common among young women. Also, affluent young adults have more time for golf, tennis, gardening, and other outdoor activities and, unless precautions are taken, they are certain to develop more wrinkles during their middle and later years.

In addition to the usual latent damage to deeper tissues, intense sun exposure will cause one immediate change in the skins of some young adults. About 25 percent of all women in the child-bearing age-group will develop, at one time or another, a bluish-brown darkening of the face known as *chloasma*. This condition is caused by the appearance of excess pigment in certain well-defined areas. Pregnancy and birth-control pills both make it worse. In the days before the Pill it was known as "the mask of pregnancy" and was considered to be a sure sign that a woman had borne a child, although this is not necessarily so. The severity of chloasma varies from a faint increase in pigment over the cheek bones to a very marked discoloration covering much of the face. The sharply contrasting light and dark areas make chloasma a cosmetic disability of the first rank, and one that is difficult to disguise with makeup. Women often find that only one weekend in the sun will change a chloasma from mild to severe and that, after this, even short periods of exposure seem to cause intense darkening.

Since chloasma is so common among young women, special precautions regarding sun exposure are necessary. In addition to wearing a hat, use of one of the benzophenone sunscreens is advisable any time the skin is exposed to the sun more than briefly. These screens are particularly effective in preventing the darkening caused by chloasma. Solbar and Uval are two representative brands containing benzophenone screens. These products are also quite suitable for the woman not subject to chloasma, since they are very effective in protecting the skin against the deep damage that causes wrinkles. Every young adult should keep a benzophenone screen close at hand, particularly during the summer, and apply it liberally to the hands as well as the face and neck. This will help prevent the unattractive pigment spots or "liver spots" that sometimes start to appear on the hands, even at this age. In spite of the name, these spots are not caused by the liver, or even remotely connected with the state of its health. (The treatment of pigment spots is discussed in Chapter VIII.) Those who feel they have to have a tan of some kind should invest in one of the "quick tans," "indoor tans," or "bronzers." Bear in mind, however, that these products will not protect against the sun unless they also contain a chemical sunscreen.

The exposure to other environmental hazards, such as wind, cold, and pollutants, is probably somewhat less at this time of life, since the young woman spends more of her time indoors. During cold weather, however, the heated indoor air is almost devoid of moisture. It is also frequently filled with the fumes of cleansers, sanitizers, insecticides, and room deodorants, and untoward reactions to all of these things do occur. Indoors, the face and hands are also exposed to heat radiated from the stove or oven, and bathed in steam arising from a boiling pot or a sink full of dishes. These are the minor hazards that everyone tends to ignore, but this is a mistake. They are all rather easy to anticipate and avoid, and exposure to them should be minimized whenever possible.

The skin of the young adult still contains enough oil to attract and hold a considerable amount of dirt, so cleansing is very important. This is particularly true if the individual has larger-than-normal pores with a tendency to become clogged. Every young adult should cleanse the face twice a day with soap. This means real soap and not a detergent bar, which is a bit too harsh for the skin of this age group, and not a superfatted soap, which is too weak. The superfatted soaps are the ones that claim to moisturize the skin or are advertised as containing cream or lotion ingredients. A common characteristic of these superfatted soaps is that they are all diluted with noncleansing ingredients, such as lanolin or cocoa butter. Consequently, they can't cleanse as well as full-strength soaps, and the young adult skin always needs full-strength cleansing power. Other common noncleansing soap additives include the deodorant chemicals and the perfumes used in bath soaps. Deodorant chemicals don't belong on the face, but the temptation is always strong to pick up a bar of deodorant soap that has been conveniently left in the bath, and cleanse the face. This temptation should be resisted at all costs. The Christmas gift soaps, with the heavy fragrances that linger on the skin, should likewise be avoided. Ivory, Lux, and Camay are three brands of true soap having none of these drawbacks. All of them will cleanse the face of the young adult with equal efficiency, but Ivory probably has a slight edge because it's unperfumed, contains no coloring agent, and is the least expensive. However, these soaps may still not provide enough cleansing for the young adult who suffers from extreme oiliness and a tendency to blocked pores. Here, one of the superfatted detergent bars, such as Dove, may be useful. Products like this dry the skin to a greater degree, and the young adult should revert to regular soap when the oily tendency has disappeared.

When using any soap, the skin should be wet with tepid water, a lather made in the hands, and then briskly rubbed into the skin. Although soap is the ideal cleanser for the young adult, it can irritate the delicate facial skin if it is used incorrectly. Therefore, no more cleansing should be done than is absolutely necessary. Every young adult should be aware of the time involved in cleansing, and the entire routine should last no longer than sixty to ninety seconds. Afterward, the skin should be thoroughly rinsed with at least three changes of tepid water. This is all that's necessary, in spite of what you may hear. One cosmetic company recommends rinsing several dozen times when using their soap, but this is ridiculous. Either the soap in question isn't very rinsable, or the company feels that their customers need some form of occupational therapy. Many beauty consultants recommend splashing the face with cold water following cleansing. This serves no purpose whatsoever, and any notion that it closes the pores or benefits the skin in any way should be discarded.

After cleansing with soap and rinsing, the skin should be wiped morning and night with a cotton pad or ball saturated with alcoholic freshener. This' adds an extra cleansing dimension to the routine which is very necessary at this age. The alcohol removes the last traces of excess oil from the skin and deep-cleans the pores. Any freshener containing a sufficient amount of alcohol is adequate for this purpose, but you would be well-advised to make your own. (See Chapter V.) It often surprises people to learn that alcohol is the only active ingredient in fresheners and that the vitamins, herbs, fruit and vegetable juices, etc., are just window dressing.

Young adults with some degree of premature dryness, or a mixed oily-dry skin, often make the mistake of cleansing their faces with something other than soap. This may be a rinsable cream or lotion, or even a nonrinsable cleanser that is tissued off. They do this on the assumption that soap aggravates the dryness. This is certainly not the right solution to this problem, because improper cleansing of the skin at this age may lead to worse things than dryness. You will frequently hear the opinion expressed that soap is too drying for the majority of young adults, but this is not true. If a young adult is intolerant to soap, there is usually some cleansing mistake at fault, such as using a detergent instead of a true soap, or overcleansing the skin in some way. Another practice that sometimes contributes to soap intolerance is using the wrong kind of MP film following cleansing, usually one that is too light to moisturize the dry skin. For the young adult who actually does have a dry skin problem, and is not making any cleansing or moisturizing errors, there are still adjustments that can be made in the routine that don't involve giving up soap. For instance, the morning freshener may be omitted entirely. This abbreviation of the routine is perfectly safe, because dry skins are less dirty and hence need less cleansing. As a last resort in conquering this problem, the evening freshener can also be omitted, but the young adult should never give up soap under any circumstances.

Every young adult should make it a rule always to have an MP film of some kind covering her skin at all times. The only exception to this would be the few minutes required to perform some other part of the beauty routine. Beginning at this age, an MP film should be the skin's constant companion throughout the remainder of life. This is because the moisture-holding ability of young adult skin is gradually declining, and unmoisturized skin is always more sensitive and vulnerable. In addition to moisturization, the skin also needs something to shield it against the attack of such things as cold, wind, and pollutants. A heavy MP film is generally not necessary at this age, only a light one worn constantly. It needn't be expensive or complicated; either—just a light lotion during the day to serve as a makeup base, and something slightly heavier at night. The Vaseline Intensive Care Daily Facial Moisturizer seems to furnish all of the moisturization and protection young adults need, and it also functions well as a makeup base. A light lotion of this type should always be applied to the face and neck *before* the makeup. Young adults generally wear more makeup than adolescents, and this is a good time to get into the habit of never wearing a colored foundation next to the skin, even if it has moisturizing properties. The pigments and powders in makeup can act as irritants in some instances, so the skin should always be protected in this fashion.

After cleansing the skin with soap and freshener in the evening, a thin film of heavy mineral oil should be applied and left overnight. This is available as Heavy Mineral Oil U.S.P., and is also sold under the brand name of Nujol. Most people have a tendency to use entirely too much of this oil, sometimes to the extent of becoming repellent to both themselves and their close friends. The secret lies in not using too much. A few drops spread evenly over the face and neck is enough to give a very effective MP film, and it won't detract from the appearance at bedtime. You might keep in mind the fact that a half teaspoon of heavy mineral oil has about the same moisturizing power as two tablespoons of most lotions.

Makeup supposedly improves the color and texture of every woman's skin, but this is more a matter of opinion than established fact. There is a small minority of women that rebels against makeup on purely esthetic grounds, and many of their male companions have a similar opinion. There is a tendency among these freethinkers to regard makeup as a sort of cosmetic panic button, something to be used only in case of a major beauty disaster. The reasoning here is that no cosmetic chemist in the world can duplicate the subtle color tones and texture of the unadorned skin, and that a few minor imperfections don't detract in the least from the overall appearance. I must admit that they do have a point. To many men, the natural woman, without makeup, is infinitely more sensuous than anything created by aritifice. But women in our society are conditioned almost from birth to wear more makeup than they need, and this has been so for thousands of years. Makeup was doubtless a necessity for ancient civilizations, unacquainted with modern skin care, but there is certainly no reason for the extreme dependence on makeup that exists among many women today. Why indeed should any young adults wear heavy makeup unless they have major beauty flaws? Most women of this age who wish to use makeup might well limit themselves to nothing more than lipstick, a little powder, and perhaps some mascara. Even these are anachronistic, reminiscent of ancient customs that refuse to die. A thousand years from now, some anthropologist studying our culture will shake his head and smile in amusement, wondering why the strange rite of making up the face persisted for so long. The answer is very simple, and inscribing it in stone might save him some digging. Millions of dollars in advertising created a want where there was no need.

But being realistic, it would be almost impossible to convince the young adult who wears makeup to use any less of it, much less discontinue it altogether. So wear it if you must, but stick to simple makeup that is moderately priced, and always apply a little less than you think you need. This advice follows from the problem of clogged pores to which many young adults are still susceptible. A little makeup is obviously easier to remove from the pores than a lot, and the simple, inexpensive makeups generally contain lesser concentrations of potential irritants, such as the pigments and powders found in all makeups, and the dispersing agents necessary to keep these substances evenly suspended. There is even a medical name for the phenomenon of pore blockage and blackheads caused by irritation from makeup. It is called the *comedogenic effect.* This is a widespread and serious problem on which a great deal more research needs to be done. If anyone past adolescence continues to have pore blockage and blackheads, her makeup is always a prime suspect.

There is another form of personal adornment, the wearing of earrings, that is sometimes associated with a more serious hazard. If a woman decides to have her ears pierced, and purchases a pair of earrings, the store where the purchase was made will often pierce the ears at no extra cost. In some instances, the buyer may also get a free case of hepatitis, caused by improper sterilization of the instruments used to do this minor operation. A woman who wants her ears pierced should be very particular about the method used to do it. The safest is a spring-operated gun that shoots a prepackaged sterile piece of metal through the ear lobe. With this approach, there is less chance of contamination by unclean instruments. In any case, the operation (minor as it is) preferably should be performed by a doctor, and never by a friend or oneself!

Like the skin, the hair of the young adult may also be past its prime: not quite as thick or lustrous as it once was, and also somewhat less resilient. It is important that all young adults be aware of this change and learn to care for their hair properly.

Hair-loss problems are very prevalent among women of this age. A severe loss often occurs three to six months following childbirth, but this always reverses itself spontaneously, and the hair eventually returns to its full thickness. Many young women experience diffuse hair-loss after stopping birth-control pills, but this also corrects itself in time. Other internal abnormalities can cause hair-loss problems that are more persistent, such as thyroid disease, and the thyroid should be the first thing checked in cases of hair loss where there is no recent history of childbirth or taking birth-control pills. But sometimes even a physician can't tell what is causing a particular woman to lose large amounts of hair. Heredity seems to play a part in many losses of this kind. Women never become completely bald, as men do, but the hair may thin to the point where it is extremely sparse and the loss difficult to conceal.

Any young woman who has a hair-loss problem, or even one who isn't blessed by nature with thick hair, should be extremely careful about subjecting it to heat and the various forms of mechanical trauma mentioned in Chapter V. She should wear her hair short, keep the style simple, and always use blunt combs with large teeth and brushes made of animal hair rather than synthetics.

Chemical damage due to waving solutions, bleaches, dyes, tints, and hair-straighteners is often a problem at this age. (I have come across few young adult women who do not use at least one of these things.) The use of chemicals on the hair not only causes a decrease in quality, but it can also contribute to a hair-loss problem by weakening the hair shaft to the point where it is easily broken off during styling procedures. Damaged hair is not only physically weaker than undamaged hair, but it is also dry, brittle, and lifeless, and has split ends. In addition, it usually lacks body and luster, has a flyaway tendency, and is hard to control. It is unreasonable to ask women to stop using these chemicals altogether and, in reality, it isn't absolutely necessary. Even though one or more chemicals continue to be used on the hair, the hair quality can be kept at an acceptable level, and any loss from breakage minimized, by using one of the new products containing hair-conditioners.

A conditioner is any substance that affects the appearance or physical characteristics of hair without changing its internal structure. The terminology used to describe these products is confusing, and even the manufacturers sometimes seem to have trouble communicating with one another. In spite of this, the products themselves are very useful, and every woman who uses chemicals on her hair should have some understanding of conditioners and how they work. They not only are of great help in dealing with damaged or thinning hair, but can also be used to equal advantage in correcting other faults, such as hair that is too fine. Generally speaking, there is no other class of cosmetic products that does so many things and does them all so well. Hair-conditioners are probably the most consistently modern and up-to-date products the cosmetic industry has to offer.

There are two types of conditioners: those that untangle wet hair, imparting manageability, and those that give the hair body or "texture," making it appear thicker and imparting holding power. Substances like egg white and beer have long been used as bodying conditioners. Their performance in this capacity is relatively poor, but many women continue to use them, either for the sake of economy, or because they are unaware that anything better exists. However, the newer bodying agents are vastly superior to these earlier home remedies since they have additional abilities that enable them to repair split ends and cracks in the hair shaft. Because they tend to build up on the hair with repeated usage, they can also protect the hair during subsequent exposure to damaging chemicals. The most popular bodying agent, collagen protein, was introduced only a few years ago, and is still going strong. There are now a variety of even newer bodying agents that work as well as protein, or even better.

Although bodying agents are more versatile by far, the untanglers, such as those found as active ingredients in creme rinses, are of almost equal importance in caring for the hair. Some of the synthetic conditioners that have appeared in the last several years are hybrids: although primarily untanglers, they may also have considerable bodying ability.

As is usual with most cosmetic products, the woman shopping for conditioners must often dig beneath a thick layer of meaningless promotional terms and slogans to expose the simple facts. *Balsam* is a word used indiscriminately to refer to conditioners in general, and even those who sell "balsam" products don't seem to have a clear understanding of its exact meaning. This situation is further complicated by the fact that there is a fragrance with the same name. The term *herbal* is also used a great deal in connection with conditioners. This can be disposed of more easily, because it refers to fragrance and nothing else. The term *natural* or *natural formula* seems to be appearing more frequently these days, but this is nothing more than bait for the gullible buyer. None of these terms really has any practical meaning relative to hair care.

Both untangling and bodying agents are found in shampoos, rinseout conditioners, and setting lotions. The shampoos generally cannot leave as much conditioning agent on the hair as the other two types of products but, with this exception, all these modes of application work very well, and you can pretty much take your choice.

Before leaving this subject, it might be well to point out that acid-reacting hair rinses, such as lemon juice and vinegar, impart no conditioning effects whatever. The practice of rinsing the hair with these substances originated many years ago when all shampoos were based on soaps. These rinses were designed to remove the dulling residue soap-based shampoos may leave on the hair. Nearly all modern shampoos contain detergents, which don't leave insoluble residues, and rinsing with lemon juice or vinegar is now totally obsolete.

One very common problem among young adults, and one that isn't solved by the use of conditioners, is oily hair. The answer here is either more frequent shampooing or a change in the type of shampoo used. If you have oily hair and scalp, you might first try washing your hair every night with your present shampoo. Contrary to what many people think, this doesn't harm the hair at all. Consider for a moment the number of times you wash your hands during the course of an average day. In most instances, this doesn't hurt the hands, and hair is made of much tougher stuff than skin. So if your hair and scalp are oily enough to need a daily shampoo, don't be afraid to do it. If this approach doesn't control the problem, you need a shampoo that is more drying. Tincture of green soap, sold in almost every drugstore, often works very well.

A great deal of the science of hair care, including dyeing, has been evolved from techniques developed in the wool-processing industry. This is because human hair is very much like sheep's wool. Wool-dyeing has been an important part of the textile industry for a long time, and this is why such things as hair-coloring products and techniques are generally so advanced compared to other cosmetic products and methods. In light of this, you can understand why many dermatologists tell their patients who want healthier and more attractive hair to never do anything to it that they wouldn't do to a fine wool sweater. No one in her right mind would think of washing a wool sweater in hot water or brushing it fifty strokes a day, but hair is routinely subjected to this kind of treatment, and hardly anyone gives it a second thought.

Many women of this age find that their hands become red, rough, and dry, and seem to stay this way, regardless of what they do. This is often called "housewife's hands." The cause of this unattractive condition is overexposure to such common irritants as foods, cleansers, wet diapers, and the various other things most women handle daily. There is often the additional history of having been subject to eczema as a child, and some authorities consider this condition an adult varient of atopic eczema. (See Chapter III.) In some cases, small blisters will appear on the fingers, a sign that the condition is rapidly progressing toward *dysidrosis*, which is a skin disease that is extremely difficult to control.

If you have "housewife's hands," and there is no practical way to decrease your exposure to irritants, wearing gloves may be the only solution. However, there is an art to wearing gloves and, if you don't know how to do it properly, they can make your hand condition worse instead of better. You should first buy some white cotton gloves, then some rubber gloves a size or two larger than you need, and wear the rubber gloves over the cotton gloves. With this two-glove approach, the cotton gloves will absorb any excess sweat, which is highly irritating to skin, and they can also be washed when they become soiled. Accumulated dirt is almost as harmful to the skin as trapped sweat and, as you know, it is almost impossible to wash the cloth linings of rubber gloves.

There are several other practical points you should keep in mind if you wear rubber gloves. Try to keep the water in which you are working as cool as possible, because hot water always encourages sweating. Never wear gloves more than twenty to thirty minutes at a time. Take them off occasionally and give the hands a chance to dry, cool off, and rest. After you have finished your work, rinse the hands in cool water, dry, and apply a hand lotion. If you have a tendency to hand problems and have to wear gloves regularly, it is very desirable to decrease the number of times a day you wash your hands with soap. When they become dirty, try covering them with a hand lotion, wiping away the excess, and then rinsing under a stream of lukewarm water. This will remove all but the most stubborn dirt. In addition to helping you avoid "housewife's hands," these same measures will also keep your nails and cuticles in better condition.

Young adults are not generally as subject to the serious health problems encountered during the middle and later years. But, in spite of this statistical advantage, young adults do develop health problems and, when this occurs, they often go undetected. Poor skin color and texture, weight problems, dark circles under the eyes, and persistent blemishes are only a few of the things that can signal some internal problem. If your health is impaired in some way, changes of makeup, exercises, and other first-aid measures won't solve the problem. Help from a physician is the only answer. The importance of preventive medicine to the young adult cannot be overemphasized. From this point onward, everyone, without exception, should cultivate the habit of regular and thorough medical checkups. Good health is an indispensable ally of beauty. It makes no sense to invest time and effort in pursuing some beauty routine only to have everything nullified by an internal problem that could easily be solved by medical treatment.

Unless there is some special nutritional need, the source of the calories consumed by young adults is of less importance, since they seem to stay healthy and attractive on almost any well-balanced diet. The problem eaters and dieters who must take a multiple-vitamin supplement should avoid those products fortified with minerals unless they are pregnant and a product of this type has been prescribed by their physician. Minerals can sometimes reactivate a blemish problem at this time of life. However, packaged supplements are not the only source of blemish-producing minerals. For example, one of the innumerable fad diets currently making the rounds recommends Vitamin B$_6$, cider vinegar, lecithin and, most important, kelp. It is a moot question how the combination of a vitamin, vinegar, a fatty substance, and a variety of seaweed can affect the weight in any way, but this isn't the important point. What is important is the fact that kelp has an extremely high iodine content, and this is one of the minerals capable of causing blemishes or aggravating an existing acne condition. Even if you did lose weight on a diet such as this, exchanging the extra fat for a complexion problem couldn't in any sense be considered a good trade.

Any woman taking birth-control pills should be extremely careful about the amount of salt she consumes. Many women tend to retain fluid while on these pills, and salt can contribute to this problem. Salt use is therefore often restricted or a substitute found. Fluid retention affects the legs most severely, but it can also give the face an unattractive, puffy look. If limiting the salt intake is not effective in controlling this condition, there are prescription medications that will effectively remove excess body fluids. However, these should not be taken indiscriminately, and are usually tried only as a last resort.

Young adulthood is the time when many women first begin to have trouble with their figures. A very common problem at this age involves the accumulation of fat in the thighs and buttocks. This is sometimes called *cellulite.* The name was invented by the French, proving that they are still as adept as ever in fabricating beauty nonsense. Most of the experts in this field doubt that cellulite even exists as a separate entity, which would seem to put it in the same category as UFOs and Abominable Snowmen. The truth is that laboratory tests reveal no differences between cellulite and plain fat, even though the name, when translated, implies that some metabolic abnormality is present. But there is apparently nothing wrong with the individual fat cells; there are just too many of them. The only real distinction possessed by this kind of fat is that it becomes highly concentrated in certain areas. The cause is thought to be a hereditary predisposition to localized fatty buildup, and the treatment is the same as that for excess fat in any other part of the body. The proponents of cellulite would have us believe they invented thick thighs and big behinds, but they have only given these features a different name. Fatty buildups of this kind frequently occur in certain isolated tribes, and these deposits are often so enormous that any outside observer would consider such women's bodies deformed and grotesque. However, in their own cultures, these deposits of cellulite, fat, or whatever you wish to call them, are considered a sign of beauty. The only thing on which everyone agrees is that excess fat in these areas is extremely difficult to eliminate. Really severe cases are best handled by a physician specializing in weight control, rather than some self-appointed guru who runs a neighborhood massage parlor. In spite of what anyone tells you, diet and exercise are still the only answers to this or any other problem involving excess fat.

Pregnancy and childbirth have a number of effects, both good and bad, on the female appearance. Women often find that during the very first part of their pregnancy there is a temporary recurrence of the oiliness and blemishes they thought they had left behind. In the later stages, however, this trend nearly always reverses itself. At this time, not only do the oiliness and blemishes disappear, but the texture, color, and general appearance of the skin often reach a level of attractiveness never attained before. Many women will tell you that both their complexions and their hair never looked better than when they were pregnant. During the last few months of pregnancy, moles are likely to pop out all over the place. Many of these will regress somewhat after the baby is born, but others will remain.

The nutritional status during pregnancy is highly important. As most women are aware, the teeth can be ruined by calcium depletion, but there are dietary supplements that will help prevent this. Gaining too much weight during pregnancy can cause the stomach, thighs, and breasts to become covered with the ugly scars called "stretch marks." This is one of the many reasons why a woman should always stay within recommended weight limits when she is pregnant.

In most instances, wearing a bra has little effect on the size, shape, or appearance of the breasts. So those who prefer to go braless can do so without fear that this practice will adversely affect the breasts in any way. Nursing mothers, however, are an exception. The extreme weight of the milk-filled breast predisposes it to the kind of tissue damage that increases sagging, so a properly fitted bra is an absolute necessity for nursing mothers.

Another common aftermath of pregnancy is varicose veins. This unpleasant condition also seems to be encountered more frequently in women who gain too much weight during pregnancy. Bulging leg veins not only look unattractive but can also cause a number of uncomfortable symptoms. Supportive stockings or bandages, when combined with intermittent leg elevation, will often suppress the symptoms, but some type of surgical intervention is necessary to permanently eliminate varicose veins. The enlarged superficial veins that sometimes appear in great numbers on the legs can pose a more difficult problem than the deeper ones, even though they never cause symptoms. This is because the exposed location of these small vessels makes them highly noticeable, and women who are severely affected often avoid shorts and swimsuits entirely. Any one of the several surgical procedures for deep varicose veins may also succeed in lessening the number of superficial veins, but otherwise, they must be destroyed individually by means of an electric cautery. This is invariably tedious and painstaking, and very few physicians will undertake the job if it involves more than a few veins. This is because complete eradication of these unsightly blood vessels is an impossible task in most instances, since new ones seem to appear almost as fast as the old ones are destroyed.

The rest and exercise habits of young adults are in many cases dictated by circumstances, and are probably less under individual control than they are at any other time of life. The young adult's most pressing problem in this area is getting enough rest, which includes both physical and mental relaxation. This is because the typical young adult (especially mothers with several children) usually gets more than enough physical exercise of one kind or another. The wife who is always complaining to her husband that she is tired most probably *is* tired, even to the point of exhaustion. This, compounded with the mental stresses usually engendered by raising a family, can make any woman look considerably less beautiful than she might under other circumstances. There is no easy solution to this problem, but sometimes the situation can be improved with better planning. If it isn't too late for you personally, plan to have no more than two children, and stick by this decision. The amount of spare time available for rest and relaxation always seems to decrease in direct proportion to the size of the family. As a corollary to this, the most beautiful women tend to be those with the smallest families. If you already have a large brood of children, you will just have to plan harder and steal whatever time you can, whenever you can. Everyone, no matter what her situation, can organize each day a little better so as to free at least a certain amount of time for the rest and relaxation that are so vital to beauty.

One of the special problems most frequently encountered at this age is a face pitted with scars, the results of severe uncontrolled acne during adolescence. These pits often will fade away by themselves in time, so it is wise to wait at least twenty-four months after the acne has subsided to see how much of this scarring is permanent. Then a decision can be made as to whether or not remedial measures are indicated.

The treatment of acne pits is surgical, and consists of removing all of the outer part of the skin and a small portion of the inner part. This may be done chemically with a caustic of some kind or mechanically with a rotating wire brush or burr. The first procedure is called chemical surgery, and the second, dermabrasion. Either should be done only by a qualified dermatologist or plastic surgeon.

It is always advisable for those considering treatment of acne scars to consult at least two different physicians and discuss methods and costs with each. As a general rule, those with the worst scars will experience the greatest degree of improvement. This is why many doctors won't operate on someone who has only minor pitting. In this instance, the degree of improvement is always slight and the results are often a bitter disappointment to the patient who is a perfectionist. Never try to talk a doctor into treating acne pits if he or she seems reluctant to do it.

In cases where chemical surgery or dermabrasion are definitely indicated, either operation can cause a tremendous improvement in the appearance. Still, there are many people who are unhappy with the results for one reason or another. First, after the patient has gone through the discomfort and expense that always accompany these procedures, the depths of the pits may be only slightly decreased. In other instances, the texture of the skin does not seem as good as it was before the operation, although this often corrects itself in time. As with any surgical operation, either of these procedures may result in certain unexpected complications. The most common is either too much or too little skin pigment after healing. In this event, there is often a noticeable line of demarcation between treated and untreated areas. Another complication is enlargement of the skin's small blood vessels, giving the face a florid look. Even though the pits may be completely gone, the occurrence of any one of these complications can make the whole experience a total disaster. However, this is the exception rather than the rule, and the majority of individuals with deep pitting who undergo either chemical surgery or dermabrasion are extremely satisfied with the results.

Pityriasis rosea is an eruption thought to be of viral origin that is often seen in younger people. It is usually most severe on the torso, but will sometimes involve the face. This eruption begins as an isolated blistery lesion with a bright red border. This is known as the "mother patch." Since individual lesions usually clear in the center as the active border spreads, most people become convinced they have ringworm, and run to the drugstore for some appropriate remedy. Typically, this will have absolutely no effect on the "mother patch" and, about ten days thereafter, similar lesions will start appearing all over the body. This disease, in spite of its ferocious appearance, is entirely self-limited, which means that it will go away by itself in time without any treatment, just like chickenpox or measles. Since you can't shorten the course of *pityriasis rosea* significantly, the only goal of treatment is to suppress the intense itching. Cool starch baths are often very helpful in doing this. Put one cup of Argo cornstarch into a tub of cool water and soak for ten to fifteen minutes. After lightly patting dry, apply calamine lotion liberally to all affected areas. This remedy is inexpensive and works as well as anything in treating this condition. It may be used as often as necessary during the day. Supplementing this external treatment with orally taken antihistamines may also help lessen the itching in some cases. Keep it in mind that no one ever died of this disease or ever became really sick with it. Sometimes the worst part of the whole thing is being covered with spots that your friends may think are either ringworm or some highly contagious disease. As a matter of fact, *pityriasis rosea* looks very much like secondary syphilis, and even a physician may have difficulty telling the difference between the two. So if you are not sure, it might be wise to have a blood test to rule out this possibility.

A very large percentage of young women who consult dermatologists do so because of cystic acne. This condition is hormonal in origin. There is nearly always a history of having taken birth-control pills during some period in the past, or the victim may have previously taken one of the high-dosage pills and then changed to one of the new low-dosage forms. Cystic acne certainly existed prior to the advent of birth-control pills, but the widespread use of these drugs seems to have increased its incidence dramatically. There are two principal differences between this condition and teenage acne. The patient is always long past adolescence, and the lesions themselves seem to start deep down beneath the skin. They become hard, painful, and tender to the touch, the skin over them turns dull red, and they seem to last an inordinate period of time. Cystic acne is frequently accompanied by a marked tendency to small whiteheads.

Although the skin may be extremely oily in some cases,

and other similarities to adolescent acne may exist, cleansers
of various kinds and medicated products are of little help in
controlling this condition. Cystic-acne lesions are simply too
deep to be much affected by anything applied externally.
Consequently, there is very little to be done at home except
to avoid picking or squeezing them. The only remedy lies in
taking one of the high-dosage "estrogen-dominant" birth
control pills (unfortunately, the other kinds don't work as
well, and can even aggravate the problem in some instances). The most consistent results in controlling cystic
acne seem to be obtained with the Enovid-E brand. All birth
control pills are prescription products, of course, and you
will have to consult a physician, who will certainly want to
examine you before prescribing them.

Even after the patient starts suitable medication, it will
take three to six months for the condition to show improvement. The cystic acne may then disappear completely, or
the victim may still be subject to a few occasional lesions.
The question then arises as to how long these birth-control
pills should be continued before they can be stopped without fear of recurrence. This varies tremendously with the
individual and may be as short as six months or as long as ten
years. Many women are plagued by cystic acne well up into
their early forties. It is wise to stay on the birth-control pills
for at least eighteen to twenty-four months and then discontinue them for several months. If the problem returns, then
the medication must be reinstated. Any young woman with
severe cystic acne not only has major psychological and
social handicaps, but the disease can eventually pit and scar
the face, just like adolescent acne. There certainly may be
risks to taking birth-control pills for a long period of time,
but such risks seem slight when considered in the light of
what might occur if cystic acne is allowed to run its course.

Fever blisters are caused by a virus. They tend to attack

the skin in response to some trigger mechanism that temporarily lowers either the local or general resistance. They frequently accompany minor illnesses, and this is why they are sometimes called "cold sores." Among the other trigger mechanisms are sun, wind, and the lowered estrogen level that occurs just before a menstrual period. Some women develop these annoying lesions every month. They appear most frequently on the lips, and a huge fever blister makes one look not only unattractive, but highly undesirable. However, they can occur on any part of the body, even on the fingers and toes. The genitals are a favorite location, and fever blisters probably occur here almost as frequently as they do on the lips. They are only mildly contagious in either area, and it is difficult (but not impossible) to transmit them from person to person through direct contact. Many individuals apparently have a natural immunity to fever blisters, and never experience one.

There is no really effective treatment for fever blisters. The only thing you can do when one starts is to wash it twice a day with soap and water and then cleanse the affected area with rubbing alcohol. If there is any great discomfort, one of the local analgesics sold in drugstores for use on fever blisters may be applied. However, these lesions will heal faster if they aren't covered with a thick, greasy film of medication. Dermatologists are often asked about treatment to prevent fever blisters and, again, there is none that is very effective. Repeated smallpox vaccinations, up to a dozen of them in sequence, are sometimes tried as a prophylaxis, but instances of complete success are rare. After a number of attacks, the body builds up an immunity to the causative virus, the frequency and severity of attacks decline, and eventually they stop altogether.

Psoriasis can start at any age, but young adults are among its most frequent victims. This is a chronic recurrent disease of unknown origin. Although stress may play some part in initiating an outbreak of psoriasis, the disease is not caused by nerves, as so many people seem to think. Neither does it seem to be related to diet or any allergy problem. Although it is sometimes associated with arthritis, psoriasis does not otherwise affect the general health. However, the discomfort and very unsightly appearance of this disease can cause serious problems. The lesions of psoriasis are round, red, and covered with a thick, silvery scale. It most often starts on the elbows and knees, but any part of the body, including the scalp, may become involved. Its course is irregular, and it will often disappear spontaneously for no apparent reason. Psoriasis is one of the greatest challenges that faces medical science today. This disease may be controlled, or the skin even cleared completely, but there is always the possibility that it will return when least expected.

The only effective nonprescription remedies for psoriasis are those containing tar. There are a number of these on the market, but Mazon seems particularly effective. Dispersable bath oils containing tar are also very helpful in some instances. Balnetar is one widely available brand.

By far the most effective prescription remedies for psoriasis are the various ointments containing cortisone, but all of these must be obtained from a physician. Another, relatively new, medical technique consists of injecting a cortisone solution directly into active lesions. This is very effective in cases where the disease is not too extensive. There are also several new internal drugs used in severe cases of psoriasis that don't respond to conventional measures. These drugs can cause serious side-effects, however, and taking one of them for any period of time involves a high element of risk. If one is willing to assume this risk, the results can be quite astonishing, and the skin will usually stay clear of psoriasis as long as the medication is continued. In all instances, the patient must be kept under constant medical supervision, with frequent checks on the blood, liver, and other vital systems. Each case must be considered individually but, in the final analysis, the patient and physician must decide together whether or not the situation justifies the use of these potent drugs.

Toward the end of young adulthood, most women begin experiencing a vague uneasiness about their personal appearance, and wonder if it isn't time to start putting forth a little more effort. That time has indeed arrived, because, like it or not, middle age and all that it implies is just around the corner.

VII Middle Age
(PSI 13-17)

This is an age of contrasts, the dividing line between those who still retain beauty and those who are rapidly losing it. Women who have consistently made beauty mistakes in the past will find that this is the time when the chickens come home to roost—or maybe "crow" is the more appropriate bird in this instance, since it is crows' feet that traditionally begin to appear at this age. In contrast to this, women who have given themselves good care over the years will often seem to have gained, rather than lost, beauty. For those who find themselves fading, this is obviously a time for stringent measures. But even those who are entering middle age with their beauty still intact can't afford to relax, even for a minute.

The skin of the middle-aged woman is rougher, thicker, and appears less translucent than that of the young adult. The pigment of the face and hands is considerably increased, and this may give the complexion a blotchy look. Localized pigment accumulations or "liver spots" often appear on the hands at this age, and sometimes on the face, too. Due to a further decline in oil-gland function, fewer of the skin's natural moisturizers are present, and there is nearly always some problem with dryness, especially during cool weather. In addition, middle-aged skin is less able to hold moisture, even during warm weather, when it is present in abundance. For the first time, the cellular buildup at the skin's surface has progressed to the point where it causes visible changes. This not only contributes to the skin's coarse appearance, but it also makes the pores look larger. The skin becomes more sensitive at this age, and at times even the simplest things seem to irritate it.

While the outer part of the middle-aged skin is becoming progressively thicker, the inner part is doing just the opposite: becoming thinner. These changes are primarily due to environmental damage, once latent, now starting to become manifest. Wrinkles of moderate depth appear about the eyes and on the forehead, due to early degeneration of the skin's ground substance. Shallow wrinkles around the mouth and on the backs of the hands may also begin to deepen at this age. Furthermore, the skin's elastic fibers are beginning to break apart, and this accentuates all the natural folds and creases. It causes the skin under the chin to be slightly droopy, and the lower eyelids may become baggy. These tendencies to wrinkling and sagging may be exaggerated by a shrinking of the facial fat-pads, which usually begins at this age. The blood vessels in middle-aged skin are nearly always enlarged, sometimes to the point where the complexion has a ruddy look. The lips are paler and thinner, and a distinct mottling often occurs on the sides of the neck at this age. This is caused by a combination of pigment increase and blood-vessel enlargement.

From the standpoint of physical and mental health, middle age is a time of transition. The hormone level is declining in all women of this age, and the tendency to gain weight is increasing. The body's needs for rest, relaxation, and exercise are changing during middle age, and the emotional outlook is often quite different. It is a time for beginning new activities and adopting new attitudes. Many long-established values need to be reexamined and reevaluated at this time of life. Middle age marks the end of one lifestyle and the beginning of another, a time for shifting gears and making important adjustments to the problems that invariably appear at this point in time. Any children left in the home have reached the age of complete independence. The middle-aged woman generally has more time to devote to herself, but she often doesn't use this time to full advantage. This is unfortunate, because the face and figure of the mature woman demand more attention, as the following pages will show.

During the middle years, there is often a resurgence of exposure to environmental hazards. There is more leisure time to pursue hobbies, such as gardening, camping, or walking, where the middle-aged woman may be in direct sunlight for considerable periods. Because of the wrinkles and other skin changes that they see every time they look into a mirror, middle-aged women often become intensely interested in learning how to properly protect themselves from the environment. For the first time in their lives, they can clearly see the results of past beauty sins for which there is no absolution. Seeing this, they also realize they are not as attractive as they were only a few years ago. Women of this age are always sincere in their desire to prevent more damage and limit, if possible, the many unattractive changes that are beginning to appear. Some of them panic and swing too far in this direction, vowing never to expose themselves to sunlight again. It's somewhat like the alcoholic who wakes up in the county hospital after a severe bout of delirium tremens, wonders how she got into such a fix, and swears off booze on the spot. In this instance, however, it is not necessary to give up sunlight entirely, and live like a bat in a cave. This would preclude many desirable activities and really isn't necessary. It's all to the good, however, that so many women of this age finally become completely aware of the disastrous consequences of environmental damage and firmly resolve to give themselves better protection than they have in the past. Generally speaking, once they have made this decision, they stick to it. The only sad note is that these women didn't make this decision many years before.

Middle-aged women will accept physical protection like hats and gloves, much more readily than younger women. There are also a number of excellent chemical sunscreens in moisturizing bases that are eminently suitable for women of this age. The Swedish Tanning Secret Lotion is one brand that seems to work well, either alone or as a makeup base. On those occasions when a sunscreen in an oily base is needed, a companion product, the Swedish Tanning Secret Oil is equally effective.

Since the middle-aged skin is not as strong as younger skin, it is also more susceptible to the harmful effects of wind and extreme temperatures. Every effort should be made to protect it against these lesser, but still potentially damaging, environmental hazards. Many women of this age use water that is entirely too hot during the cleansing procedure, or become addicted to such things as facial saunas or hot towels. They do this for a number of reasons, all of them related in some way to the alarming signs that have recently appeared. Some decide that the fault lies in not cleansing thoroughly enough, and that scalding water will help open and purge impurities from their somewhat enlarged pores. Others try to stimulate the skin's circulation with heat, believing that this will in some mysterious way help to reverse aging and skin damage. Contrary to what these deluded women think, heat doesn't help the skin in any way, and can only aggravate and intensify existing problems.

A considerably drier and more sensitive skin necessitates a change in cleansing habits at this age. The middle-aged skin should be cleansed once a day with soap and freshener. This should be done at bedtime, when the dirty film covering the skin reaches its height. It would be advantageous if a woman could continue using regular soap throughout middle age, but this is not always possible, since regular soap may cause the skin to become dry and increase its sensitivity. In this case, a switch must be made to one of the milder specialty soaps, preferably one containing no perfume. The unscented Neutrogena is ideal for this age group. Even though the irritant potential of this product is low when compared with regular soaps, the middle-aged skin should not be lathered too briskly and cleansing time should never exceed sixty seconds. One advantage of Neutrogena is that it is slightly more rinsable than other soaps, but the skin should still be rinsed in three changes of water to make sure that all soap residues are removed. These residues tend to irritate mature skin, and are much more likely to form if the water used for cleansing and rinsing is hard or has a high mineral content. Those who live in areas having extremely hard water would be well-advised to keep a bottle of distilled water near the washbasin for cleansing and rinsing. Only in this way can they be absolutely certain that no soap residues are left on the skin.

After cleansing with soap and rinsing, the middle-aged skin should be wiped with a cotton ball or pad saturated with an alcoholic freshener. This should be repeated five nights a week, the other two nights being reserved for thinning, which will be discussed later. If this routine seems to cause dryness or increases the irritability of the skin in any way, the use of alcoholic freshener may be decreased from five times a week to only two or three, or even omitted entirely in exceptional cases.

Every middle-aged woman should select her alcoholic freshener with great care. These products, along with MP films and masques, are the junkyards of the cosmetic industry. The routine ingredients common to all of them, such as vitamins, proteins, and fruit juices, injure only the pocketbook. But many fresheners contain chemical irritants that can harm the skin. These are the products that claim to give a "radiant, glowing look" or "close the pores." Middle-aged women are prime prospects for fresheners like this, because they are often beginning to develop a pasty, sallow look and enlarged pores. The chemical irritants themselves are of two types, each having a different but equally undesirable effect on the skin. One type irritates the small blood vessels, and the resultant expansion causes the skin to take on a rosy color. However, frequent use of fresheners containing these chemicals may result in permanent blood-vessel damage. Those most frequently encountered are aromatic substances and essential oils extracted from bushes, trees, flowers, herbs, etc. Menthol, thymol, camphor, eucalyptol, methyl salicylate, witch hazel, bay, and capsicum are a few of the names you will find on freshener labels. The other type of chemical irritant, those that supposedly close the pores, are usually acid-reacting salts of aluminum or zinc. These were formerly called "astringents" and, fortunately, they are not as popular as they once were. All of these acid salts are weak chemical thinners and attack the outer portion of the skin, causing it to swell slightly. These irritants can't in any way close the pores, but they sometimes make them appear smaller by partially swelling them shut. The reactions caused by both types of chemical irritants violate normal physiological principles, and both should be avoided. With the help of the lists of ingredients furnished by cosmetic manufacturers in response to new labeling regulations, the consumer should be able to tell a great deal more about the contents of the fresheners she buys, and she can predict their effects with greater accuracy. Avoiding the traps contained in various fresheners is sometimes the most difficult part of caring for middle-aged skin. If you have any doubts at all about the safety of the alcoholic freshener you are now using, you should play it safe and make your own. (See Chapter V).

In the morning, the middle-aged person should use neither soap nor alcoholic freshener. She should simply remove any residual nighttime MP film with a piece of cotton saturated with lukewarm water. Those with better-than-average skins may use an alcoholic freshener instead of water if they wish, but this practice should be discontinued immediately at the first hint of dryness. If this extra cleansing in the morning causes no discomfort, then congratulations are in order, because this means that your skin is in better shape than that of many of your contemporaries.

Bathing is very apt to cause a persistent dryness and scaliness of the entire body during middle age, and some adjustments in this cleansing procedure may become necessary. Changing your regular soap for one that is superfatted will often help. Basis is a superfatted soap that has been recommended by many dermatologists throughout the years. The newer Tone soap also seems to work well. The middle-aged woman may find that a dispersible bath oil is very helpful in fighting body dryness, particularly during cold weather. During the winter, outdoor winds and indoor dry air can quickly strip the entire skin of its moisture. There are several reasons why the middle-aged woman is particularly prone to generalized dryness during cold weather. The skin's natural moisturizers become thicker when the temperature falls, and don't spread as well, so skin coverage is uneven. Also, insensible perspiration, an important alternate source of moisture during warm weather, decreases to very low levels in cold weather.

During the day, the middle-aged woman needs a product that will not only adequately moisturize and protect the face and neck, but also serve as a makeup base. One product that is satisfactory for these purposes is the Deep Magic Moisturizing Lotion. Women of this age should always apply something like this first, and any makeup should be worn over it. Never make the mistake of trying to kill two birds with one stone and dispense with the MP film just because the tinted foundation you are using claims to have a "moisturizing" base. Not only do the pigments and powders in tinted foundations sometimes irritate the middle-aged skin when placed in direct contact with it, but their presence greatly accelerates moisture loss. So you should never depend solely on these products to keep your skin adequately moisturized.

One reason cleansing with soap has such a bad reputation among the middle-aged is that they don't always apply a heavy enough moisturizer after using it. The combination of soap and alcoholic freshener has an even greater potential for drying middle-aged skin, so it's important that an MP film of adequate weight be applied immediately following cleansing at bedtime. Unscented Albolene Cream is the preferred overnight MP film for this age group. The reader may well be taken aback by the mention of Albolene, since it has been used for years as a cleanser, and a nonrinsable one at that, but it is also one of the best heavy MP films money can buy. It is a versatile product and can sometimes serve another useful purpose. If a woman happens to be using a heavy oil-based makeup, as many women of this age do, a good portion of this can be removed with Albolene and tissue prior to the regular cleansing. Cold cream, baby oil, and other nonrinsable cleansers can also be used in similar fashion to *preclean* the skin. With most of the makeup already gone, it will be much easier for the soap and freshener to remove what remains, and the use of these stronger cleansers can be held to a minimum. After the cleansing routine is completed, a small amount of Albolene can then be reapplied to give the skin a thorough overnight moisturizing. Albolene liquefies at normal skin temperatures and spreads easily. If you don't use too much the resultant film will be almost free from greasiness or tackiness. The efficiency of this or any other moisturizer that doesn't contain water can be increased by prewetting the skin for several minutes prior to application. This can be done very easily by patting the skin with wet pieces of cotton or holding a moist washcloth to the face. This prewetting is done automatically when you rinse the face after using soap, but the alcohol in your freshener will immediately extract most of this moisture, leaving your skin dry again. Hence, the desirability of prewetting if you are using both an alcoholic freshener and a waterless oil or grease as your MP film.

This is the age when many women must start thinning their skins on a regular basis to remove the accumulation of dead cells at the surface. Cellular buildup makes the skin drier and rougher, gives it a coarse look, and causes the pores to appear enlarged. The pigment contained in these excess cells can also affect the skin's color. All of these problems can be helped by thinning the skin.

One of the abrasive surface-thinners, such as a loofa sponge, should be sufficient to remove the modest amount of cellular buildup that is often present at this time of life. After rinsing away the last traces of soap, and while the skin is still moist, the face should be gone over with a loofa

sponge or other thinner, using a circular motion for relatively flat surfaces, such as the cheeks and forehead, and a
horizontal or vertical motion for contoured surfaces. Only
moderate pressure should be applied, and under no
circumstances should thinning be carried to the point where
the face becomes raw or irritated. It should be done twice
weekly, immediately following the nighttime cleansing with
soap, at the time you would normally complete your cleansing routine by using a freshener. On nights when thinning is
done, the alcoholic freshener should be omitted.

The elbows and heels often show a marked cellular
buildup at this age. These areas may become very rough and
dry, visibly thickened, and highly unattractive. In some
instances, the dry buildup at the outer edges of the heels
becomes so exaggerated that painful fissures appear. This
condition is almost exclusively confined to women and is
thought to be related in some way to hormonal decline. Both
of these areas should be softened prior to thinning by soaking in water. This can be done most easily in the bath, and
requires at least twenty minutes, or longer for the heels if
the buildup is particularly heavy. After softening, the
elbows can be thinned with a loofa sponge, but a pumice
stone works better on the heels. On leaving the tub, a film of
petrolatum or Vaseline should be applied to both areas. If
the condition is especially severe in either area, the
moisturizing effects of petrolatum may be augmented by
covering the skin with an occlusive plastic wrap and leaving
it in place overnight. With the elbows, this can be accomplished by wrapping them with rectangular pieces of plastic,
like Saran Wrap, and sealing the edges with tape placed
around the upper arms and forearms. Plastic food bags are
more satisfactory for the feet. These can be slipped on over
the feet after the petrolatum is applied and a pair of socks
worn over them. The socks will keep the plastic bags in place

during the night. You can also use this method during the day if you are planning to stay home.

Makeup problems seem to increase during middle age, and there are a number of possible explanations for this. In the first place, the skin is more sensitive at this age to all foreign materials, including those that go into makeup. This tendency is increased if the skin has suffered environmental damage or been abused in some other way. Another cause of makeup problems during middle age is the habit of using heavier makeup, which many women begin at this time due to the greater number of flaws and imperfections. Not only can this heavier film irritate the skin directly if precautions are not taken, but more cleansing is required to remove it, and this may precipitate other problems. Finally, there is always the possibility of a comedogenic reaction in those who habitually wear heavy makeup. (See Chapter VI.) The comedogenic effect seems to be more prevalent among middle-aged persons using makeup manufactured by some of the smaller cosmetic companies. The formulations of these products often deviate from established norms by a wide degree, and in other instances, production standards are not as high as those of larger companies.

It is almost impossible to recommend specific brands of makeup for the individual, because of the many subjective factors involved in its selection. It would be easier if there were any one company whose makeup not only appealed to everyone but had a perfect safety record. But no existing company even comes close to this. There are only two short and simple rules regarding the use of makeup on middle-aged skin. Always favor brands made by the larger companies and, when you have made your choice, use it sparingly. In your search for suitable and safe makeup, keep in mind the fact that it is designed primarily to hide or deemphasize beauty defects, not to care for the skin, and that it can often create problems of its own. Think of it as a necessary evil and, instead of trying to find products that are good for the skin, concentrate on finding those that will cause the least amount on trouble.

The hair undergoes a slow but steady decline in both quantity and quality during middle age, but this rate may fluctuate widely under certain circumstances. There is often a sharp increase in hair loss at the time of menopause, and any operation or surgical procedure may cause the same thing, although this kind of loss is more apt to be temporary. The incidence of hair loss from internal problems, including diseases and internally administered drugs, is higher at this age. Any hormonal therapy that includes the use of testosterone, the male hormone, can greatly accelerate the loss of hair. Since nearly every middle-aged woman has somewhat less hair than she did a few years before, it needs to be treated more gently. Excessive manipulation and hair trauma can be avoided if she keeps her hair short and adopts a hairdo that requires a minimum of styling. At this time of life, brushing, ratting, and teasing should be avoided altogether, and even rolling and setting should be done as infrequently as possible.

Damaged hair is more frequently seen during middle age due to increased exposure to bleaches, dyes and tints. In the eyes of many women, these chemicals are often more of a necessity than a luxury at this time of life, and their increased use stems from the fact that middle-aged hair has usually lost much or all of its color. In ancient times, when strands of gray began to appear, women dyed their hair black by using lead combs dipped in vinegar. The lead salts so produced combined with the hair's sulfur, causing it to turn black. The products sold today that gradually darken grey hair are based on this principle, and usually contain a solution of lead salts. All of them work reasonably well, and are perfectly safe. However, due to the limitations of this method, most women prefer to dye or tint their hair. Possibly the most common coloring mistake made by middle-aged women, particularly brunettes, is using too dark a shade.

In addition to using one of the shampoos made for bleached, dyed, or tinted hair, every middle-aged woman who colors her hair should use a creme rinse, followed by one of the setting lotions that is high in protein. This combination not only helps avoid hair loss while combing out wet hair and styling it, but improves the hair's texture and makes it appear thicker. Protein is substantive to hair, meaning it sticks to it and builds up on the hair shaft, and this coating can also help protect the hair during subsequent exposure to harsh chemicals. For the rare middle-aged woman who doesn't use chemicals, and has hair of good quality, a protein shampoo to make the hair look thicker is usually all that's necessary (Protein 21 is an effective product of this kind.)

The nails, which are structurally very much like the hair, may also begin a decline during middle age. They often become dry and brittle and show an increased tendency to split and separate. This is the reverse of what you might expect, since the middle-aged woman is generally doing less housework and contacting less irritants than younger women. But the middle-aged nail is weaker and much more susceptible to such things as nail polishes, cuticle-removers, nailhardeners, and artificial nails, all of which can contribute to nail and cuticle problems. Cuticle-removers contain strong alkalis and often cause separation of the nails. If the cuticle is kept pushed back with an orange stick and clipped as needed, it is usually unnecessary to use these products. Nail hardeners contain formaldehyde. They cause not only allergic reactions but severe nail damage, which may result in the loss of one or more nails. The glue used to attach artificial nails will occasionally do the same thing.

Any woman who is experiencing nail problems should bear in mind that the nails are also more sensitive to metabolic abnormalities and various medications at this age. If elimination of all the possible external causes doesn't result in improvement, then the problem is very likely internal and a thorough physical examination is indicated. Incidentally, the protein nail-builders used by many middle-aged women are ineffective, regardless of the source of the problem.

The state of the general health has an increasing influence on beauty as the years go by. Women who have avoided their family doctors for a number of years will often react to a pronounced loss of beauty by shrugging their shoulders and saying that it was bound to happen sooner or later. Some of the more energetic and affluent may flee to one of the expensive and exclusive spas that prey on insecure women, but these can offer little more than cosmetic solutions of a temporary and superficial nature. In reality, neither approach seems very intelligent if there is a possibility that the problem is due to hormonal imbalance, disease, or nutritional deficiency. The only proper reaction to a greater-than-expected loss of beauty during middle age is to visit a physician as soon as possible.

A physician can also be of invaluable help to the middle-aged woman in another area: that of weight control. Obesity problems are even more likely to occur at this age than earlier, and can seriously affect the general health by putting a strain on the heart, blood vessels, and other internal organs. This is why the middle-aged woman who is fat can't expect to retain beauty for very long. Overweight women will invariably try every kind of fad diet before seeking professional help. This is because everyone, from their milkman to their hair stylist, seems to have a dietary tip or two guaranteed to solve any weight problem. Unfortunately, following the advice supplied gratis by amateurs often complicates a weight problem instead of solving it. The correct approach to the problem of losing weight is one of the many things in life that is basically simple and straightforward but has been muddled beyond belief by those who are not fully qualified to give this kind of advice. Regardless of what anyone says, there are only two sure ways to lose weight, by eating less or exercising more. Any reducing diet should be precisely balanced to assure adequate vitamin and mineral intake and forestall deficiencies. Better results will be obtained if the details are worked out by a physician who is familiar with both your metabolism and your psychological status.

There are always a number of middle-aged women who are looking for some shortcut to beauty, and these are the ones who are always taken in by the various frauds that seem to come and go with monotonous regularity. Probably the most recent involves Vitamin E. This vitamin is totally ineffective when applied externally, and goodness knows how many carloads of Vitamin E oil have been wasted in this manner. Many people are now taking huge oral doses in the hope of improving their health and appearance. However, it was recently reported that high doses of Vitamin E may damage the blood vessels and liver and cause weakness and fatigue. This is just another of the many instances involving the misuse of vitamins. It has always been extraordinarily difficult for the average person to put these substances into proper perspective and realize that, although the body does need a certain minimum daily allowance of each vitamin to carry out its metabolic functions, any excess introduced into the system acts like a foreign substance and is potentially toxic. We are still getting, and certainly will continue to get, other unpleasant surprises along these lines. Some of the toxic effects of megadoses of Vitamin A are described in Chapter V. Although documentation is scanty, there is an indication that high doses of Vitamin B12 may also cause undesirable changes in the skins of some women.

The excesses of an unregulated life can detract from beauty at any age, but their effects on the middle-aged individual are particularly noticeable. Many people of this age don't sleep as well as they should, and suffer from chronic fatigue. This makes them more susceptible to anxiety and other forms of nervous tension. Another source of these and the other nervous problems so prevalent at this age is situational changes. The most important is the new lifestyle that suddenly materializes once a woman is freed from the burdens of raising children. However, for reasons that are still obscure, what should be a change for the better often marks the start of a middle-aged woman's deterioration. From the standpoint of beauty, the secret of a successful psychological adjustment to middle age seems to lie in a high level of both mental and physical activity. This includes all sorts of occupations, hobbies, diversions, and interests that use both the mind and the body. Constructive mental activity promotes relaxation by banishing the stresses, anxieties and tensions of middle age, and this enables the individual to rest better. Physical activity not only has a similarly beneficial effect on the quality of rest, but a number of subsidiary benefits. It imparts a sense of physical well-being, helps prevent weight problems, and seems to help prevent the deterioration to which the inactive individual is so prone at this time of life. These are some of the reasons why sustained mental and physical activity are so important to health and beauty throughout middle age. The middle-aged woman who finds herself with time on her hands should acquire a hobby, take a course, become active in some organization, participate in a sport, or start an artistic endeavor. The exact types of activities aren't as important as the fact that the person is doing things that will simultaneously occupy and stimulate both the mind and the body.

Rosacea, a special beauty problem of the middle-aged, is a disease of the oil glands characterized by severe inflammation and infection. It primarily affects the large oil glands of the nose, but those of the cheeks may also be involved, and occasionally a few lesions are even seen on the chin and forehead. It is similar in appearance to teenage acne, consisting of elevated blemishes that may contain infected material. The inflammation surrounding these lesions and subsequent blood vessel enlargement causes the skin to appear bright red. Also like adolescent acne, rosacea is in some way tied to the hormone balance but, in this case, the level is declining rather than rising. In long-standing cases, the nose may become considerably enlarged. Rosacea and its attendant "rum blossoms" were once thought to be a sure sign of alcoholism. Although alcohol can sometimes make this disease worse, it is often seen in teetotalers. Rosacea is bad enough for a man's appearance, but for a woman it is a beauty catastrophe of major proportions.

Diet definitely seems to affect this condition; however, the degree varies greatly depending on the individual. All victims of rosacea should give up coffee, tea, and alcohol, and cut their consumption of sugar to a minimum. There are also reports that hot, spicy foods tend to aggravate rosacea, so these should be similarly avoided. Externally, the affected areas should be washed with soap and water at bedtime and some type of medication applied. Good results are often obtained with Sulforcin lotion. After this is removed in the morning, the regular skin-care routine may be followed during the day. Rosacea does not seem to be aggravated by makeup.

If these measures don't result in improvement, the help of a physician must be sought. As with adolescent acne, antibiotics constitute the basis of the medical approach to the treatment of rosacea. In some instances, supplementary treatment with hormones causes improvement. In severe, intractable cases, where the nose has become disfigured, the removal of excess tissue and restoration of the nose to its natural contour is nearly always indicated.

During middle age, the inelastic tissues in various parts of the body may be unable to retain the skin's normal resiliency, and the pull of gravity causes extensive localized sagging. In addition to environmental damage, heredity and stretching of the skin during some period of rapid weight gain may play a part in causing this condition. The unattractive results include drooping upper eyelids, baggy lower eyelids, loose skin under the chin, pendulous breasts, a sagging abdomen, and sagging thighs and buttocks. There is no way of correcting these conditions yourself. Facial and body exercises, massage, and diet produce little or no improvement. However, a competent plastic surgeon can correct any one or all of these conditions, literally remaking your body from top to bottom. These surgical procedures require hospitalization, and the discomfort, expense, and difficulties tend to increase as you work your way down the body. The eyelid operations are the simplest, and the ones involving the breasts, abdomen, thighs, and buttocks the most difficult. In these last three areas, there is often a localized fat problem that increases the sagging. Any of these operations may be done separately, but when the buttocks are repaired, the localized fatty bulges on the lateral aspects of the thighs are usually done at the same time. The removal of excess tissue in these two areas is known as the "riding breeches" operation.

The methods used to correct localized sagging were almost unknown to the public until a few years ago, but things are different today. At the time of this writing, there is a movie playing locally that depicts a woman who simultaneously undergoes all of these operations during her stay at a clinic in Switzerland. After a degree of restoration usually reserved for vintage Rolls Royces of the rarer kind, the job is completed, and she emerges from the hospital in mint condition.

To be absolutely candid, any one of these operations involves some very serious surgery. As a form of insurance, you should always insist that anyone you allow to remake your body be a member of the American Board of Plastic and Reconstructive Surgery. There are many surgeons capable of doing these operations who are not members of this group, but you will be a little safer with one who is. There is nothing wrong with shopping around beforehand, especially when the risk and expense are of this magnitude. You wouldn't think of adding a room to your house without getting bids from at least two or three builders, and this is a comparable situation. So if you are considering one or more of these operations, you should get a professional opinion and estimate of the total cost from at least two plastic surgeons. You may find that both the opinion and cost estimate vary with different surgeons, not because of any differences in degree of competence, but because individual surgeons always employ slightly different techniques and, as one finds with any group of independent contractors, some are able to run their businesses more efficiently than others and can offer you a lower cost.

At this time of life, many women notice superfluous hair

appearing in places where it is definitely unwanted and never grew before. All of the body hairs become stiffer and heavier with age, and the upper lip and chin may become covered with coarse bristles. Also, a mat of fine downy hair may appear on the cheeks during middle age, which bleaching may or may not camouflage. Although there is a hereditary predisposition to superfluous hair, the precipitating factor is the ascendancy of adrenal over ovarian function, tipping the balance in favor of the male hormones. There are four methods of removing excess hair: shaving, depilatories, waxing, and electrolysis. However, only the last three need concern us here.

Depilatories contain strong chemicals that remove hair by eating through the shaft. The popularity of these products seems to wax and wane. During times when they are popular, dermatologists see many adverse reactions to them. Depilatories should never be used on the face. Even on the legs, they should be discontinued immediately at the first sign of irritation.

Wax is intended for the removal of fine downy hair. Although it can be purchased and used at home, this is one procedure that can always be done better by a beautician or cosmetologist. In these cases, the excellence of the results is well worth the extra cost. In a salon, the area to be treated is first covered with melted wax. Then strips of cloth are pressed into the wax before it hardens. These strips serve as handles to facilitate removal of the hardened wax, which is always peeled off in the direction of hair growth. The only drawback to waxing is that the hair must be allowed to grow long enough to be grasped and held firmly by the wax. This is one reason why shaving and depilatories are far more popular.

Electrolysis is the treatment of choice for darker hairs that cannot be removed with wax. This method is usually impractical for the legs, but it can be used to remove unwanted hair on almost any other part of the body. It is generally safe, and the majority of operators are competent. Skin damage from electrolysis is exceedingly rare. A few chin hairs can be removed in one session, but a mustache or other heavy growth may require a dozen sessions or more. In these cases, it would be wise to get an estimate of the number of sessions required and the approximate cost before beginning treatment.

Some patients become discouraged because the operator will have to go back over areas where hair was removed, perhaps several times. This is not because the operator missed hairs during a previous session, but is due to the fact that some of the hairs were in a resting stage and not visible at the surface. The operator must keep going over an area until all these dormant hairs have been removed. Although some people develop a rather intense irritation around the hair follicle from electrolysis, the only real complication of any consequence is infection. This often requires that the patient be put under the care of a physician for appropriate therapy. Infections following electrolysis can sometimes cause pitting, just as acne does, so you should seek medical help if there is any intense irritation or sign of infection following this procedure. All in all, electrolysis is a very worthwhile beauty aid, and people are apprehensive about it only because they don't understand it. There are few beauty procedures that attack a problem so directly and generally give such outstanding and satisfactory results.

In middle age, most women experience some superficial wrinkling around the eyes, forehead, and mouth. However, in other instances, almost the entire face becomes covered with a fine superficial wrinkling. This is caused by extensive degeneration of the supporting tissue or ground substance of the skin's inner portion, due primarily to environmental damage. This condition can be treated by either chemical surgery or dermabrasion. (See Chapter VI.) As mentioned previously, these operations are done by both dermatologists and plastic surgeons. In addition, superficial wrinkling is treated by many cosmetologists by means of a modified form of chemical surgery. When this operation is done by nonmedical personnel, it is often called "skin peeling" or "skin layering." Most authorities agree that it is risky to allow people who do not have medical degrees to do these deep-thinning procedures. Certainly some cosmetologists are competent to perform chemical surgery, but many are not. To be perfectly safe, a prospective client would have to have a great deal more information regarding a specific cosmetologist's abilities than is available to the person who merely answers an advertisement or takes a friend's recommendation.

To satisfactorily correct superficial wrinkling, all of the skin's outer portion and part of its inner portion must be removed. Although done primarily to correct the wrinkling, there are some valuable secondary benefits to the middle-aged skin. All of the cellular buildup is removed along with the skin's outer portion, the pores are unblocked, and excess pigment and pigment spots are removed, along with any rough, red spots that have formed on the surface. When the outer portion of the skin regrows, it has lost its coarse, leathery look, the pores appear smaller, and the color is more even. The most important effect, of course, is the plumping-up of the skin that occurs as the inner portion heals. This causes a marked decrease in the degree of wrinkling. After either chemical surgery or dermabrasion, a month or two may pass before healing is complete and the redness has subsided to the point where a person looks presentable. It may be four or five months before the maximum benefits of these procedures are realized Certain areas, like the upper lip, don't respond as well as others, and localized touchups may be necessary to achieve the full degree of improvement possible with these operations.

The question most frequently asked by those considering treatment for superficial wrinkling is how long the results will last. The answer is anywhere from one to ten years, but this time varies tremendously in individual cases. Any lasting effect is very much dependent on exchanging the bad beauty habits that caused the superficial wrinkling for good beauty habits that will help preserve the new tissue.

Although an allergy can be caused by any product applied to the skin or hair, deodorants, soaps, shampoos, hair dyes, and makeup are most frequently involved. Among the other products that also produce allergies are nail polishes and miscellaneous nail products, hair conditioners, perfumes, and hair-removers. Cosmetic allergies vary in severity from mild redness and irritation of the skin or scalp to acute swelling and blistering of these areas. The thin skin of the ears, face, neck, and backs of the hands is particularly susceptible, and the eyes may be swollen shut by a particularly severe reaction. This is the general picture seen in all cosmetic allergies, regardless of cause. It is sometimes difficult to distinguish between allergic reactions and irritative reactions that are not truly allergic. The most common irritative reaction is the intense scalp-inflammation and hair-breakage that accompanies the improper application of waving solutions, bleaches, or hairstraighteners. In mild cosmetic allergies, the treatment consists simply of avoiding the offending product and letting the allergy run its course. In severe cases, particularly where the eyelids are involved, medical help may become necessary. The treatment here is the same as that for poison ivy, or any other allergy of external origin, and involves the systemic administration of cortisone.

The most important part of solving any allergy problem is identifying the offending product. In many instances, the location of the reaction will give a clue as to which product is involved. Lipsticks affect the lips, deodorants and antiperspirants the underarm area, and hair-removers the legs. Nail-polish is an exception in that it will often affect the eyelids, rather than the nails or cuticles. In those instances where the cause is less obvious, the diagnosis cannot usually be made without testing the skin to suspected products.

Most of the time, you can do this yourself. All you need is a box of plastic bandages or Band-Aids. The technique is as follows: Apply a drop or equivalent portion of the product to be tested to the gauze part of the bandage and place it on the inner surface of the upper arm. Check the skin underlying the gauze portion of the bandage after twenty-four hours to see if there is any redness or blistering. If there isn't, it should be left in place another twenty-four hours. When the bandage is removed at the end of forty-eight hours, if the area of skin underlying the gauze is perfectly clear, you are not sensitive to that particular product. If there is any degree of redness, you probably are sensitive to it and, if there is blistering, you most certainly are. With this technique, any type of makeup can be tested, such as your foundation, blusher, powder, mascara, eye shadow, liner, and lipstick. Other types of products, such as sunscreens and MP films, can be tested in exactly the same way. You can also test yourself to other more irritating products, but all of these should be applied directly to the skin of the arm and left uncovered. If you are doing more than one of these open tests at the same time, it helps to outline the test area in ink, so that you can tell where each one was placed. The test areas are checked at twenty-four and forty-eight hours, as with the closed tests, and read in the same way. Nail polish can be painted directly on the skin. Hair-removers, deodorants, antiperspirants, and perfumes are generally tested using the open method. Soaps, shampoos, and other cleansers can also be tested by this method, but they shouldn't be applied to the skin full-strength. They must first be diluted with water to a concentration of 2 percent. In other words, one part of the product is mixed with fifty parts of water to make the test solution. A drop is then applied to the skin, allowed to dry, and then read at both twenty-four and forty-eight hours. Testing cosmetic products with an extremely high irritant-potential usually requires special dilutions and techniques, and these are best done by a physician.

Finding the offending product is helpful but gives no indication as to which specific ingredient caused the trouble. Consequently, switching to a similar product in another line may not solve your problem, since products with similar uses frequently have ingredients in common, even when made by different companies. However, as a result of the new cosmetic labeling regulations, the allergy-prone individual can now identify the specific ingredients contained in all cosmetic products, and this may offer some help along these lines.

When a physician tells a woman she is sensitive to a specific product, one of the most frequent reactions is, "I couldn't be sensitive to that; I've used it for years!" However, the length of time a product has been used is of little consequence in deciding whether or not an allergy exists. One of the most basic principles of allergy is that a reaction *never* occurs on the first exposure to a substance, but only after a number of exposures. The length of time it will take an allergy to build up to the point where a violent reaction occurs varies anywhere from a few days to a lifetime; therefore, a product that has been good to your skin for a number of years may suddenly attack it without warning.

The subject of the next chapter is the later years. This time of life is traditionally associated with the end of beauty, and is still regarded by many women as a hopeless situation as far as personal attractiveness is concerned, something to be endured as patiently and philosophically as possible. This passive attitude may have been justified at one time, but it certainly isn't today.

VIII The Later Years
(PSI 18-20)

It is theoretically possible for any woman to be beautiful throughout the entire span of the later years. There are two ways this can be accomplished: either by practicing good beauty care throughout the earlier years, or by spending a considerable portion of the later years in the company of dermatologists and plastic surgeons. These two alternatives are so predictably related to one another that they may almost be put into a mathematical equation. This equation would show that the woman who has made a lifelong effort to preserve her beauty will have very little need for professional help during the later years. Unfortunately, it would also show that the woman who has neglected this care will be almost completely dependent on these professionals throughout the remainder of her life.

The skin in the later years is delicate, like that of a child, although the weakness is due to age and damage, rather than immaturity. It further resembles the skin of a child in that it is very dry, sensitive, and easily irritated. It is also noticeably rough to the touch and various growths may be scattered over its surface. The pigment accumulation in the skin's outer portion reaches its zenith at this age. The dark pigment spots that were once confined to the hands now appear on the face, and stand out very noticeably, even against the more heavily pigmented background. Due to cellular buildup, the whole outer portion of the skin is much thicker than it was during middle age. This not only causes the pores to appear enlarged but it tends to block them. Small blackheads and whiteheads begin to appear, even though the oil glands are small and sluggish. Although the hair of the body and scalp undergo widespread attrition at this time, the amount of superfluous hair on the face and neck shows a marked increase.

In contrast to the skin's greatly thickened outer portion, the inner portion is much thinner and greatly weakened, due to the fact that the supporting ground substance is shrunken and degenerated and the elastic fibers broken into tiny pieces. This causes a marked increase in wrinkling. There is extensive sagging, particularly of the jowls, neck, and eyelids. All of the skin's natural folds are exaggerated, and deep lines appear for the first time. The lips become progressively thinner, and the borders are indistinct. The blood vessels show further enlargement. Due to the skin's extreme thinness, they become much more prominent and may even appear to be "broken." The facial fat-pads may almost disappear at this age. This not only accentuates all of the wrinkles and lines, but gives the countenance a gaunt, bony look.

The most significant internal event of the later years is the almost complete cessation of ovarian function. Much of the dryness and loss of texture in older skin can be attributed to this depletion of circulating female hormones. Even more striking is the masculinization that many women undergo at this age, due to the continued secretion of male hormone by the adrenal glands. (A comparable degree of feminization occurs in older men.) The male and female identities, once so distinct, begin to merge during the later years, and the boundaries separating the sexes become blurred.

Physical health, or lack of it, plays an increasingly large part in determining beauty during the later years. Nearly every older person suffers some slowing of the metabolic processes, and all are more subject to degenerative changes and chronic diseases.

One result of the marked physical and psychological changes that occur at this age is that although the older person is easily fatigued, she often has extreme difficulty sleeping. The mental and physical activities in which this person has either the opportunity or ability to participate vary widely, due to the great individual differences in both motivation and general health. The later years are often punctuated by situational changes of far-reaching consequence, resulting in a completely different lifepattern. The married woman often spends some or all of this time as a widow, and this is only one of the many sociological adjustments she must face during her later years. It is sometimes difficult for women to maintain their enthusiasm for beauty when confronted with all this, but an interest in the appearance can be of inestimable psychological value to older women. At this age, the search for beauty is often a greater reward than beauty itself.

There is probably less exposure to environmental hazards during the later years than at any other time of life. Even when this occurs, the consequences of exposure are quite different from those of earlier years. This doesn't mean that protection from the sun isn't important during the later years, because it is, but for a somewhat different reason.

The chief concern prior to this time was the latent damage caused by solar penetration of the skin's inner portion. Now, however, the thickened outer portion of the skin and its pigment act as a natural sunshield. This barrier greatly decreases the amount of solar radiation that gets through to the skin's inner portion. Furthermore, if deep damage does occur at this age, the latent period between the time of the damaging event and the end result, such as more wrinkling, may be greater than the individual's life expectancy. So, with habits of less sun exposure, built-in protection, and the possibility of not living long enough to pay the price of her carelessness, the older woman may not be quite so concerned about deep skin damage. But sunlight is still harmful to the older skin, because it seems to stimulate all of the rough red spots, molelike growths, and pigment accumulations that appear on the skin's surface. These often respond to any intense sun-exposure by rapidly increasing both in size and number. Consequently, adequate sun protection is essential for every older woman who indulges in outdoor activities.

There are many benefits associated with activities of this kind, older people enjoy them, and such outings should be encouraged. Before leaving the house, however, every older woman should equip herself with a hat, a pair of gloves, and a chemical sunscreen. Eclipse is a relatively new sunscreen product that gives excellent protection. It also comes in a moisturizing base that is suitable for older women and can be worn under makeup. Women of this age rarely use sunscreen products with oily or greasy bases but, if one is needed, the Bain de Soleil Suntan Creme, recommended for children, will work equally well on their grandparents.

The only other environmental hazard of any importance at this age is dry air. This is very hard on a skin that not only has difficulty holding moisture, but is almost devoid of natural moisturizers. Older people invariably set the thermostat too high during winter, and hot, dry air can quickly dehydrate older skin. Room humidifiers are often helpful in solving this problem or, in lieu of this, open pans of water placed about the living quarters may provide an impromptu solution.

The skin during the later years is cleaner than at any other time of life. There is not only less actual exposure to dirt and pollutants, but these undesirable substances are less likely to be attracted to the drier skin. Although less cleansing is needed, the extreme dryness and increased sensitivity of the older skin sometimes make it intolerant to even the most superficial cleansing. This can cause problems, and working out a suitable cleansing routine for the older woman is often a process of trial and error. At this age, the skin should be cleansed only once a day, preferably at night. Fresheners containing alcohol are too drying and should not be used at all by older persons. Those whose skins are in better-than-average condition may be able to continue using one of the milder soaps, such as Neutrogena. Conversely, if the skin is in poor shape, almost any soap is likely to cause increased dryness and sensitivity and make the skin uncomfortable. Before giving up soap, however, the older person should always try to make some adjustment in the routine that would enable her to continue using it, at least on a part-time basis. Less lather can be applied, the skin rubbed less briskly, and the cleansing time decreased to thirty or forty-five seconds. If this doesn't solve the problem, soap should still not be abandoned on the spot, but tried, say, on a twice-weekly basis.

In this case, some other cleanser must be found to replace soap the other five nights of the week, or even used exclusively if this limited use proves impractical. The cleansing product most suited to this situation is a rinsable lotion. The choices are very limited here, but one brand that seems to do a good job is Pond's Creamy Lemon Facial Cleanser. The heavy lemon fragrance is unfortunate, because it doesn't add a thing to the product's cleansing ability, and may even cause it to disagree with some people. Regardless of what it says on the label, any product of this type should always be rinsed off with water after cleansing, never tissued off. If the older person consistently removes a rinsable cleanser with tissue, and never rinses with water, the residue will eventually irritate the skin and increase its dryness and sensitivity. This bad cleansing habit also encourages the appearance of large pores and blackheads.

Rinsable cleansers are milder than the mildest soaps, and those using them can take a little more time during the actual cleansing procedure than they ordinarily would. However, these cleansers don't mix with water as well as soaps, and this means they are more difficult to rinse from the skin's surface. Removal can be facilitated by first going over the face and neck with a washcloth wet with lukewarm water, and then rinsing the skin with the usual three changes of water.

If you are using a rinsable cleanser nightly and the skin still remains somewhat dry, resist the temptation to use oils, greases, creams, or any other kind of nonrinsable product for cleansing. These just won't get the skin clean, and all of them invite problems. Using a heavier moisturizer following cleansing will often solve this dryness problem and make the skin feel more comfortable.

Among rinsable cleansers, there are many that claim to moisturize the skin. These should be avoided, as should all cleansers that promise to do any more than remove the skin's dirty surface film.

Bathing problems, such as extremely dry skin and flakiness, are common at this age, and the older person should use only the mildest of bath soaps. Neutrogena Baby Soap seems to work well as a bath soap for older people. In addition, a dispersible bath oil should always be used in conjunction with this or any other kind of soap. During cool weather, those with very dry skins may also find it necessary to apply a body lotion following the bath. Bathing with soap every day doesn't agree with some older skins, and in these instances, the frequency must be decreased to two or three times a week. On the days soap is not used, the body may be covered with a dispersible bath oil before entering the tub or shower, and the oil rinsed away with water. This doesn't get the body as clean as soap, of course, but it's certainly preferable to not bathing at all. There are actually some women, usually of advanced age, who can't tolerate soap under any circumstances, and must rely entirely on this method.

The skin's need for the moisturizing benefits provided by MP films increases throughout the later years, and the older skin requires the heaviest of MP products. It also does better with the simple, uncomplicated ones that are kind to older skin. The heavy MP films used by older persons are sometimes called emollients. After any residual night-time MP film is removed in the morning with a cotton pad wet with tepid water, one of the heavier lotions or creams should be applied to the face and neck. The Jergens Facial Moisture Cream works well as a combination daytime MP film and makeup base for older people. Any makeup applied should be worn over the MP film, because such products as tinted foundations are particularly hard on older, more sensitive skin. After bedtime cleansing, the use of a very heavy product is desirable, so that the older skin can be completely moisturized overnight. Here, any brand of petrolatum, such as the familiar Vaseline, is the product of choice. Petrolatum is the heaviest MP product available at any price. It is the ultimate moisturizer. Since it contains no perfumes, preservatives, or any other irritants of older skin, it causes no problems, even when left on for prolonged periods of time. Unfortunately, this product is so thick that it is difficult to apply a film that is thin enough to be cosmetically acceptable. Melting the petrolatum before application is sometimes helpful. This can be easily done by putting a small amount in a tablespoon and holding a lighted match under it for a few seconds; then a thin film of the warm liquid can be applied to the face and neck. Thick films of petrolatum are esthetically unpleasing, as well as unnecessary.

Promotion of MP products to this age group by various cosmetic concerns is sometimes indistinguishable from a three-ring circus. Meaningless jargon of a quasitechnical nature abounds in this area, some of it palpably deceptive, and all of it designed to make the potential buyer think that some expensive cream or grease has very potent therapeutic powers. Generally speaking, this sort of fraudulent promotion increases in direct proportion to a product's price and, with the most expensive ones, it borders on the ridiculous. In some instances, these products contain non-moisturizing ingredients that are not only useless but possibly harmful to older skin. Two of these ingredients, hormones and mild chemical thinners, are heavily promoted to women of this age.

The hormones used in MP films include estrogen, progesterone, and pregnenolone. All of these may have some slight plumping effect on the skin, but they don't accomplish this through moisturization. Rather, they do it by changing the metabolism of the skin's living cells, causing them to swell. This effect is not only unpredictable from person to person, but brought about by means that are contrary to the natural processes of human physiology. Also, it has never been proved that applying hormones to the skin year after year is entirely safe.

The practice of putting mild chemical thinners into MP films is relatively new, but no less deplorable. Urea and allantoin are the two most frequently found. They do make the skin feel somewhat softer, but don't contribute a thing to genuine moisturization. The price the skin must pay for this slight improvement is increased vulnerability to all sorts of problems. Many older people find their skins are irritated by products containing these chemicals and cannot use them at all. If you haven't tried them yet, you can do your skin a favor by continuing to ignore them completely.

Older skin should be thinned twice weekly, and this should always be done during the interval between cleansing and application of nighttime MP film'. Thinning helps remove the excess of dead cells that have accumulated at the skin's surface. The thinned skin is not only more attractive but more easily moisturized. This procedure also helps unclog the pores and removes small blackheads, so it is particularly valuable to the older skin with pore problems. The main thing to keep in mind while using a thinner of either the abrasive-surface or abrasive-particle type is that older skin is extremely delicate. Consequently, any thinning procedure should be done with great care, and the skin subjected to somewhat less pressure than would ordinarily be applied. Otherwise, the procedure is exactly the same as described in the previous chapter, even to the extent of using the same kind of thinner, a loofa sponge. The particle type of thinners sold to this age group, such as those containing soap grains, almond meal, and pumice, are disappointing on several counts. Not only do these particles lack abrasive power, but the bases used to contain them are usually unacceptable in one or more respects. They are either non-rinsable, like cold cream or, in cases where they are rinsable, the base contains a soap or detergent. Even when used cautiously, any particle-type thinner in a cleansing base may prove too drying for the older skin.

Among the other thinning products sold to older women under various pseudonyms are the clarifying, exfoliating, sloughing, or peeling lotions. These invariably contain a chemical thinner of some sort and often have a high alcoholic content. Both chemical thinners and alcohol tend to be incompatible with older skin and can cause it to become dry, irritable, and extremely sensitive. These products closely resemble the medicated lotions used by adolescents. The chemical thinners found in them include salicylic acid, resorcin, and sometimes milder ones like urea and allantoin. The older person should avoid all preparations of this type, no matter what they are called. If thinning is indicated, the abrasive route is always much safer than the chemical, and it also does a better job.

It often seems that the list of extravagant, ineffective, and useless products sold to those of this age is inexhaustible. However, there is only one more group of products corresponding to this definition that is of any importance. These are the so-called masques or facials, used not only by this age group, but by all others, and usually for the wrong reasons. These products are sold for a variety of purposes, such as cleansing, moisturization, and thinning, but actually, they don't provide any of these to any practical extent. Masques can be divided into rinse-off and peel-off types, the former being the more common. The rinse-off masques are usually based on mineral clays, gums, or proteins, and come in hardening and nonhardening varieties. Nearly all rinse-off masques have some minimal cleansing ability, and the ones that harden often place the skin under enough tension to affect its small blood vessels. The swelling this causes has a plumping effect on the skin and may temporarily improve its appearance. This phenomenon is sometimes called the "masque effect." It is harmless enough if achieved solely by mechanical means, but many of the rinse-off masques do it through the inclusion of some of the same chemical irritants found in fresheners. (See Chapter VII.) Masques containing these chemicals should be avoided, as their continued use may damage the skin's small blood vessels.

Peel-off masques all dry or harden, and most of them are capable of causing the "masque effect" without resorting to chemical irritants. For this reason, they are probably the safer of the two types. Peel-off masques are generally based on rubber, wax, or plastic of some kind. Many of these thin the skin by adhesion, meaning they may pull a few dead cells from the skin's surface as they are removed. Their effectiveness in this respect is extremely low when compared to abrasive thinners.

The subject of masques and their uses and limitations has always been surrounded by a vast amount of misinformation. They are often sold for moisturizing the skin but, strangely enough, this is the thing they do least. The majority of them don't even contain moisturizing ingredients and, therefore, are physically incapable of raising the skin's moisture level. Rinse-off masques usually have no moisturizing ability at all, and the few peel-off products that are occlusive enough to conserve moisture suffer from the handicap of time, meaning that they are not left in place long enough to cause any real change in the skin's moisture content. If someone touts the moisturizing value of a masque, pay no attention, because any MP film can moisturize the skin as well or better than a masque, not to mention more economically.

Rinse-off masques may have made some sense years ago as cleansing aids, when the use of nonrinsable cleansers was more widespread. Otherwise, cosmetic masques don't have—nor have they ever had—much value as bona fide beauty aids. However, they are still going strong in some quarters. The "organic face lifts" advertised in the newspapers usually turn out to be nothing more than rinse-off masques based on protein, usually with a dollop of herbs, vitamins, or fruit juices. Sometimes these masques are warmed before application or used in conjunction with vibrators or some other kind of appliance, but none of these adds a thing to the masque's overall effect. The sellers of these concoctions claim they will rejuvenate the appearance and even remove lines and wrinkles without surgery. This kind of malicious puffery might be laughable if only it didn't delude and disappoint so many older people. Just for the record, face-lifts always come out of operating rooms, not jars.

The use of makeup varies considerably among older women. Some apply it very heavily, while others use none at all. Heavy makeup would certainly be easier to justify at this age, because older women do have more beauty defects, and properly applied makeup can be most helpful in disguising them. The sunken cheeks, the increased prominence of the nose, the deep lines on the face, and the disappearing lips—all these flaws can be minimized with the proper use of makeup. The most frequent mistake made by older women is applying makeup with too heavy a hand. What is most often needed is a little more finesse, and a little less makeup. In this instance, a session with a professional makeup consultant can be invaluable, and this is something every older woman should be encouraged to do. Cosmetic companies frequently send their top consultants on tour, and many of these individuals are very talented.

Selecting specific makeup products is apt to be more of a problem in later years. The older woman is likely to find that many makeup items feel uncomfortable on the skin or disagree with it in some way. Since cleansing heightens the skin's sensitivity, many of the makeup problems encountered at this age are initiated or reinforced by bad cleansing techniques. This is most likely to happen if a woman wears heavy makeup that requires considerable cleansing to remove. In this instance, the method described in the previous chapter for preliminary removal of heavy makeup with nonrinsable cleansers and tissue can be of great value. With this technique, less actual cleansing with soap or rinsable cleanser will be needed and, as a result, the skin should be less sensitive and feel much more comfortable.

Nearly every older woman has a hair-loss problem of some proportion. The hair becomes sparser with age. It is usually dry, brittle, and lifeless. Beyond this, there are the more severe hair-loss problems caused by glandular abnormalities or internally administered medications. A drug used in the treatment of high blood pressure had to be taken off the market several years ago because of its many side effects, one of which was causing the hair to fall out, even to the point of complete baldness in some cases.

Women of this age who feel they are losing their hair often develop the habit of constantly pulling or tugging on it. Some may do this unconsciously. Others do it to demonstrate their problem to friends and acquaintances and show them how easily the hair is removed from the scalp. The loss in these cases may be real or it may be purely imaginary, but in either event the hair shouldn't be continually abused in this manner. The important thing to determine in situations like this is whether the rate of hair loss is remaining steady or gradually increasing. There is need for concern only if the rate is increasing, because this often indicates an active disease process of some kind. A simple test to determine this can be made by combing the hair out, using an equal number of strokes, over a towel at the same time every day. A daily count is kept of the number of hairs found on the towel and comb for six weeks and, if the count increases over this period, there is a good chance that the problem is of a progressive nature. Under these circumstances, a medical checkup is definitely indicated. If this reveals no scalp disease or internal abnormality, the next step is to give the hair a vacation from mechanical trauma, heat, and chemicals. (See Chapter VI.) If these measures fail to halt the hair loss after a reasonable period of time, a woman must accept the fact that she is losing her hair and neither she nor anyone else can do much about it. However, women rarely become completely bald, regardless of the problem's source.

Once a woman has accepted an irreversible hair loss, the emphasis obviously changes from the therapeutic to the cosmetic. The easiest and most effective cosmetic solution is to invest in a wig. These are in no way harmful to the remaining hair and can be worn indefinitely without the slightest risk. If this approach is not satisfactory for some reason, measures can still be taken to help preserve and emphasize whatever hair is left. Most importantly, the hair should not be washed more than once a week. This limitation is dictated not by any harmful effects inherent in the shampoo itself, but solely because the hair is weakly attached, and untangling, drying, and styling it may remove more. One of the conditioners containing both untangling and bodying agents should be used after every shampoo. This not only helps avoid pulling the hair out, but the bodying part of the conditioner will make the hair look thicker after it is dried and styled, giving the overall appearance of more hair. Even when using a conditioner, the hair should always be blotted dry with a towel instead of being rubbed, and treated very gently during the untangling and styling.

One of the most frequent problems in later years is separation of the nails from their beds. Why this happens is not known, although it is much more likely to occur if a thyroid condition is present, and particularly if a woman is taking thyroid medication. Certain nail products, such as cuticle-removers, nail-hardeners, and artifical nails also aggravate this condition. Occasionally there is separation of all ten fingernails but, fortunately, loss of the entire nail never occurs.

The only thing that seems to benefit nail separation is avoiding water in any form and keeping the nails as dry as possible. This is very difficult to do; however, many older women have their hands in water a great deal more than is necessary. They often wash them up to a dozen times a day, sometimes due to an unconscious germ phobia, and sometimes just out of habit. After bathing or any essential hand-cleansing, the undersides of the fingernails should be wiped with a cotton swab dipped in rubbing alcohol. This helps remove the last traces of moisture from beneath the nails. Rubber gloves retain moisture and should never be worn by anyone whose nails are separating. Gelatin by mouth is of no value whatsoever, in either preventing or alleviating nail separation or, for that matter, in any other nail problem.

Any relatively sudden change in the appearance at this age is more likely due to some health problem, rather than an error in the beauty routine. Blood, liver, kidney, and glandular diseases are frequent at this age and can quickly destroy beauty. A woman who is in the habit of having checkups on a yearly basis should consider increasing this frequency to twice a year. The harmful effects of many internal conditions are often irreversible, so early diagnosis and treatment are extremely important.

Older people traditionally have poor appetites. As a consequence, they are more subject to nutritional deficiencies. These often contribute to the dryness, scaliness, and inelasticity found in older skin. Tissue destruction always tends to outrun tissue replacement during the later years, so a diet high in protein is indicated. Some unsaturated fat in the diet is also desirable, as well as an abundance of fruits and vegetables. The older woman is more subject to mineral depletion and should always supplement her diet with a multiple-vitamin product fortified with minerals.

There are rarely any weight problems during the later years, because the chronically obese have long since succumbed to heart attacks and strokes. As you have probably noticed, there are very few fat octogenarians to be seen anywhere. At this age, there is more trouble maintaining fat than getting rid of it. The facial fat pads, which are so vital to the appearance, normally become smaller with age, even in the absence of any chronic diseases or nutritional problems. Every woman of advanced years should try to keep her weight at a constant level, but this isn't always easy. Nature seems to conspire at this time of life to tear down all of the tissues, including fat, bones, and muscles. This is why good nutrition is so essential during the later years.

Miraculous potions to restore youth and beauty are heavily promoted to people of this age, but older women will save themselves a good deal of disappointment if they will accept the fact that all of these are worthless and, in some circumstances, dangerous. You should never take by mouth or allow yourself to be injected with any chemical or extract of animal origin that is in any way controversial. Some legitimate treatment to restore beauty may be developed some day but, until that time comes, the older woman shouldn't allow herself to be used as a guinea pig by unscrupulous quacks.

Keeping mentally and physically active throughout the later years is an absolute prerequisite to beauty. Nevertheless, the increasing psychological and physical problems toward the end of life often limit these activities, sometimes severely. The older person may need the encouragement of family or friends to maintain habits that will benefit both health and beauty. Exercise and other regular physical activities are certainly of tremendous value here, but nothing is more precious to the older woman than a mind that is receptive to new ideas and welcomes new experiences.

Of all the special problems that affect older persons, shingles is one of the most serious. This disease is caused by a virus, and the characteristic skin-eruption that accompanies it is caused by a viral attack on certain nerve roots. The cause is in no sense psychological, or due to nervousness. The symptoms of shingles may begin several days, or even weeks, before the eruption appears, and consist of pain or some other unpleasant sensation along the course of the nerve under attack. The first skin lesion is usually a red spot similar to an insect bite. Other spots then appear in quick succession, and become surmounted by blisters filled with a yellowish fluid. This represents the height of the eruption and, from this point, it gradually subsides, the blisters being replaced by thick, adherent crusts. The average duration of shingles from the appearance of the first lesion to complete healing is about three weeks. The disease may leave in its wake some deep and unsightly scars. In addition, the nerve-inflammation may persist for months or years after the skin is healed, causing excruciating pain.

Although the trunk is the most frequent site of attack, shingles often appears on the face, and the resultant scars may be very difficult to hide with makeup. One characteristic of shingles is that it never occurs on both sides of the body at the same time, always being confined to either the right or left. If an eruption extends much beyond the midline of the body, the odds are that it isn't shingles. There is no known preventive for this disease other than avoiding children with chickenpox and those persons known to have been exposed to it. This may sound strange, but the shingles and chickenpox viruses are very similar, and some investigators believe that one is an attenuated form of the other.

Once the signs appear, there is very little in the way of self-treatment that will halt the process. Taking aspirin for the pain and applying ice packs to the affected area may give some relief, but neither will affect the progress of the disease in any way. The blisters should not be opened under any circumstances, as this invites infection, which can greatly increase the scarring. In all instances, early treatment of shingles by a physician is highly desirable. The usual treatment consists of giving cortisone, either by mouth or injection. This is very helpful in suppressing the inflammation and will usually shorten the course of the disease. With early treatment, both the scarring and pain that accompany shingles can be held to an absolute minimum. In any case of shingles affecting the forehead and upper eyelid, there is always the possibility of eye involvement, severe eye damage, and even blindness. Consequently, a specialist in eye diseases should be consulted any time shingles strikes an area near the eye.

Generalized facial sagging is a sign of extensive destruction of the skin's elastic tissues. This causes the skin to become loose and hang in folds, and deep lines to appear. The pull of the facial muscles on weakened skin often contributes to the development of this condition, and the absence of fat pads deepens the lines and increases folding. The treatment for diffuse facial sagging is colloquially known as a face-lift, and it lies entirely within the realm of plastic surgery. There has been so much written in the popular press about this particular operation that there can hardly be a literate woman who isn't familiar with it. A recent article in a national women's magazine not only gave a detailed description of this operation, but estimates of costs in a number of cities and the names of recommended plastic surgeons in each. However, the preliminaries leading to a face lift and what happens afterward are often of more importance than the operation itself.

For those in need of a face-lift, there are two main barriers: one financial, and the other psychological. A woman shouldn't necessarily abandon the idea just because her means are limited, but should visit one or more plastic surgeons in her area and discuss fees. Plastic surgeons as a group are neither more nor less charitable than the rest of mankind, but they are usually willing to discuss ways of holding costs to a minimum for patients in reduced circumstances. On the other side of the coin, many women who can well afford this operation cannot bring themselves to accept it, even though they need it in the worst way, feeling that a desire for plastic repair marks them as frivolous or denotes some other character defect. This is a foolish point of view. Having plastic surgery denotes no more of a warped personality than using makeup does. The difference between the two is only a matter of degree, not basic principle.

If these obstacles are overcome and a woman elects to have a face-lift, she should always keep her expectations within reasonable bounds and realize that neither her physical appearance nor her life-situation will be changed as much as she might like. In other words, she won't look like a Hollywood starlet, and the people who didn't love her before the operation won't love her afterward. Plastic surgeons are becoming more adept at weeding out the unstable personalities who would actually suffer psychological harm from a face-lift, rather than being helped by it. These are generally people who have some unresolved mental problem and expect a face lift to change everything; they often develop severe mental aberrations or otherwise go off the deep end when it doesn't. Since the object of a face lift is to make the patient look better, not drive her crazy, a greater effort is being made to identify and eliminate persons who react in this way.

The only esthetic drawback to a successful face lift is a slight loss of expression or immobility of the face, giving it in some instances a faintly unnatural look. This is usually of minor importance, however, compared to the degree of overall improvement. The effects of this operation will last on the average from three to five years. The exact time depends to a large extent on the quality of care given the skin during subsequent years. With good care, the time may be extended considerably; with bad care, it almost certainly will be shortened. Probably the most important thing a woman can do to preserve her new face is to zealously protect it at all times, especially from such things as sun, wind, and extremes of temperature.

Pigment spots, warty moles, and rough, red spots are the three types of benign growths that appear during the later years. Although any or all of these growths may be removed during the course of chemical surgery or dermabrasion, it is more usual to have them treated individually by a dermatologist.

Pigment spots are in many ways the most difficult of the three to treat successfully. The trick is to remove them without causing any appreciable scars. Unfortunately, there is no externally applied product, either prescription or nonprescription, that is even moderately effective in lightening these unattractive lesions. However, sun exposure always darkens them, so the use of an appropriate sunscreen can be helpful in arresting their progress. Dermatologists treat these dark pigment spots by three methods: burning them, applying caustic chemicals, and freezing. Since each pigment spot may require several treatments, the removal of multiple lesions may be a lengthy and painful process. Those on the backs of the hands are more difficult to treat because of the thinness of the skin, and some dermatologists won't treat them at all in these areas.

Older people will sometimes develop an incredible number of warty moles. These begin as light brown spots that grow slowly and gradually become elevated. The end result is a large, dark, cauliflowerlike lesion with a warty surface that sometimes measures half an inch in diameter. Some of these look frightening, but none is really dangerous. Susceptibility to these growths is determined in part by heredity and, in many cases, there is a history that the parents or grandparents of the victim had them. Women often wait until they are literally covered with these molelike growths before seeking help. Only a few can be removed during each session and, since new ones continue to appear, getting rid of them entirely is almost an impossibility. Women often seek help for the first time when one of these growths has become hung on clothing or a piece of jewelry, and the top split or partially torn away. In this state they can easily become infected. Nearly any oil or grease will soften these growths and smooth their surfaces, but this has little effect on their deeper portions and cannot remove them.

The larger lesions must be excised surgically; the smaller ones can be removed by burning or freezing. However, the method most commonly employed by dermatologists is to apply an anesthetic spray and simply peel these growths off the skin surface with a curved knife called a curette. With this method, up to a dozen of these warty growths can be removed during an office visit. If you have one or more of them, they should be watched closely and removed if they become larger than one-quarter inch in diameter. By doing this, you can avoid the permanent scars that often result from the removal of larger growths.

The rough, red spots that appear on older skin are generally more numerous on the light-exposed areas, such as the face, ears, and hands. They come in many sizes and shapes, varying from discrete conical horns that may stand an inch or more above the skin surface to large, red scaly spots several inches in diameter. The average lesion seen in most dermatologists' offices is no more than one-eighth inch in diameter and appears as a rough, red, slightly elevated spot with a hard top. Actively growing lesions usually exhibit some degree of sensitivity or tenderness. The only home remedy for these spots is plain castor oil, massaged into them twice daily. This won't completely eradicate rough, red spots, but it will soften and remove part of their hard tops so that they will look better and feel more comfortable.

These growths are precancerous and should be completely removed by a physician at the first sign of activity. Some of the same methods employed to eradicate pigment spots are used here, including burning, the application of caustics, and freezing. These lesions also respond to X-ray and may be thus treated alone or in combination with some of the previously mentioned methods. There is also a prescription chemical, 5-fluorouracil, with which the patient may be able to remove superficial lesions at home

The smaller growths leave little or no scars when they are removed, but the larger ones destroy tissue and can leave some very ugly scars. Consequently, early diagnosis and treatment are desirable in all cases.

The development of cancer represents a final stage in the skin's destruction and degeneration. There are two kinds of skin malignancies, basal cell cancer and squamous cell cancer.

The basal cell cancer is the less serious of the two, since it grows by local extension and does not spread to distant parts of the body through the blood and lymphatic systems as do other malignancies. Basal cell cancers occur most frequently on the face, ears, and neck. They typically appear as elevated pearly nodules or shallow bleeding sores on the skin's surface. These cancers are often deceptive in that they grow slowly, and older women will often defer treatment of these lesions indefinitely, hoping they will heal of their own accord.

The squamous-cell type of cancer is much more dangerous and will eventually spread to other parts of the body if left untreated. This occurs most frequently on the hands and lower lip. The initial lesion is a small, hard lump that rapidly increases in size, sometimes forming an ulcer in the center. All cancers of the squamous-cell type should be given immediate attention. They are usually treated by either surgery or irradiation, but sometimes a combination of the two is necessary. Just because a cancer starts in the skin, rather than the cervix or breast, doesn't mean it's any less malignant or can be taken less seriously.

Both basal and squamous-cell cancers destroy tissue, sometimes at a very rapid rate. A small scar is the best you can expect if you develop one of these malignancies, even though it receives prompt treatment. If one is allowed to progress, you may lose an eye, an ear, the nose, a lip, or even your life. So don't fail to seek professional help if any rough, red spot or lump on your skin changes in any way. Skin cancers are the ultimate result of beauty neglect. They are also the ultimate destroyers of beauty.

The next chapter is devoted to the beauty industry, and all those folks who state unequivocally that their product or service will make you beautiful. It would be foolish to accept all these claims at face value, but it would be equally foolish to slam the door before taking a look at what they have to sell.

IX Products and Practitioners

The beauty business is comprised of the cosmetic companies who make the products, and the beauty operators, such as cosmetologists, beauticians, estheticians, and cosmeticians, as they are variously called, who provide beauty services. Of the two, women are more dependent on the cosmetic companies, who provide the products they use daily. Since beauty services are discretionary in nature, they are used by a much smaller portion of the population. However, both these segments of the beauty industry have much in common, and their identities even merge occasionally. It is not unusual to find manufacturers operating beauty salons and, conversely, many salons also offer their own private-label cosmetics.

The beauty business is absolutely unique, and a source of neverending fascination to those who have studied it in depth. It is a mixture of pharmacy, fashion medicine, and theatrics, a strange blend of the modern and the archaic, the logical and the illogical, and the useful and the totally useless. All these components are so intertwined and commingled that it is almost impossible for a nontechnical person to make distinctions between products and services that have value, and those that are a complete waste of time and money. The purpose of this chapter is to try to put all of this into perspective, and separate the wheat from the chaff or, more appropriately, the top sirloin from the baloney.

I was once discussing the cosmetic industry with the beauty editor of a woman's magazine. She asked me why I always pooh-poohed the practice of using ingredients like royal jelly in skin-care products. I told her it was for the same reason I would pooh-pooh the use of aspirin in the treatment of leprosy if anyone ever suggested it. I concluded by saying that if Ingredient or Medication A had never been reported by a reliable source to have some favorable effect on Condition or Disease B, putting A into products used to treat B made no sense. This story, I think, illustrates very well the fact that the cosmetic industry still relies heavily on "miracle ingredients" and other such nonsense to sell many of its products.

As a matter of fact, the cosmetic industry of today is very reminiscent of the drug industry at the turn of the century, when cure-alls for every human affliction were hawked on street corners and advertised in newspapers. If the drug industry had made as little relative progress as the cosmetic industry over recent years, consumers would still be at the mercy of the snake-oil salesmen and vegetable-compound vendors, and without antibiotics and the other life-saving drugs they now have.

Some insights into the reasons for this discrepancy may be gained by taking a look at the companies themselves and those who are responsible for their essential character and direction. Many are managed by supersalesmen or supersaleswomen, with little or no scientific background. Research and development often consists of nothing more than attempts to duplicate a competitor's successful product or changing the physical form, packaging, or perfuming of an existing product in order to stimulate sales. In addition to some pretty weird products, the results of all of this include a good deal of inaccurate label copy, volumes of deceptive and misleading advertising, and very high prices. However, this is all slowly changing, and the time is past when you could take a face cream developed by your gypsy grandmother, package it, and make a fortune. There is no doubt that the cosmetic industry will eventually catch up with the drug industry and the rest of the world, and that the quality and effectiveness of all beauty products will be vastly improved over what they are now.

But the average woman can't afford to wait for this beauty millennium, and this is why products that are both effective and reasonable in price, and available now, have been sought out and mentioned in this book. In addition to these, there are many other excellent products that have not been mentioned, due to limited availability, or for any one of a number of reasons not directly related to effectiveness. I also realize that not every reader will like all my personal choices, or be able to integrate each and every recommended product into her individual beauty routine. In some instances, the fragrances may not be appealing, while in others the product may not be compatible with the reader's favorite makeup. There will also be a few people who are actually allergic to some of these products. Furthermore, any one of them may be discontinued unexpectedly, and it is almost a certainty that at least one or two recommended products won't be available by the time this book is published. This is because the cosmetic industry is traditionally preoccupied with trends and fads. As a consequence, its products enjoy relatively short lives, and tend to come and go in rapid succession.

If a recommended product doesn't suit you, doesn't agree

with you, or isn't available, you will obviously have to find a replacement. The first part of this chapter is devoted to a discussion of beauty products in general, the purpose of which is to help you evaluate products other than those specifically recommended by brand name. With this information, you should be able to seek out and recognize effective beauty products without having to rely entirely on brands. There will also be some additional background information on how to utilize beauty products for maximum benefits, and how some of the new developments, such as those affecting product labeling, can work to your advantage. In addition, some alternate products, which you might find useful, are mentioned by brand name.

All of the sunscreens recommended throughout this book are based on only three types of chemical ingredients: PABA, the PABA derivatives, and the benzophenones. Other acceptable chemical sunscreens include homosalate, cinoxate, menthyl anthranilate, digalloyl trioleate, and triethanolamine salicylate. The average screening ability of these is somewhat lower than that of PABA, the PABA derivatives, or the benzophenones, but the relative potency of individual sunscreens isn't the only factor in determining whether or not a product will adequately protect you. The concentration of sunscreen in the product is of equal, if not greater, importance, and this information isn't always stated on the label. To further complicate matters, some of the sunscreens containing alcohol or water undergo a reduction in effectiveness when they are applied to the skin, due to the evaporation of these volatile components.

There are several general principles regarding sunscreen usage that can be derived from these facts. First, all sunscreens should be applied liberally, regardless of their active ingredients or physical form. If a sunscreen product dries on the skin, which means it contains either water or alcohol, you should always apply a second coat. When using any product containing one of the less potent sunscreens, either a very thick initial coat or several coats should be applied. This means that, from a theoretical standpoint, you can use almost any sunscreen you wish and still receive maximum protection, provided you apply a sufficient amount. In a sense, it is the user, rather than the manufacturer, who makes the final determination of a sunscreen's effectiveness or lack of it, and the adequacy or inadequacy of the protection against sun damage.

The most common complaint women have about sunscreens concerns their compatibility with makeup. There is usually no problem when using such simple products as a light film of powder, but even liquid makeup can be ruined by an underlying coat of some sunscreen product. This is particularly true during the summer when the combination of heat and perspiration seems to catalyze dormant incompatibilities. The greatest number of complaints come from young adults using Solbar and Uval. This is unfortunate, because these screens are particularly useful to this age group. The other sunscreen products recommended for use under makeup seem to cause fewer problems. These include PreSun, Swedish Tanning Secret Lotion, and Eclipse. Another sunscreen that seems to have good makeup compatibility under most conditions is Maxafil. This product contains two of the less potent sunscreens, but both of these are present in relatively high concentrations, and it offers good protection.

There is no pat solution for incompatibility problems. Wearing as little makeup as possible and experimenting with sunscreens in different bases may eventually produce a winning combination for you and the particular makeup you feel you can't do without. Another approach is to try one of the sunscreen products that contains makeup. The opaque pigments and powders used in these combinations have a high degree of inherent screening ability, even by themselves, so the blending of chemical sunscreen and opaque material results in a product with maximum screening ability. These mixtures are similar to cream foundations. Two representative brands are RVPaque and A-Fil Cream. Unfortunately, products of this type have various esthetic drawbacks and limited cosmetic appeal. Also, they are rather heavy and the choice of shades is extremely limited. In spite of this, these products provide excellent protection during any period of intense or prolonged sun exposure. If you can find one that appeals to you, by all means use it. As a matter of fact, if you were to be set afloat on a raft in the South Pacific for a month, this is the type of product you should take.

Most sunscreens have some moisturizing ability, and this ability increases as you go from the lotions to the creams to the oils to the greases. The specific exceptions to this are the PABA and amyl dimethyl PABA screens in alcoholic solution. Here a separate MP film must be applied over the sunscreen to prevent moisture-depletion.

Always try to match your sunscreen product to your activity. All of them will eventually wash away with swimming or heavy perspiration, but some tend to adhere better than others under these conditions. PABA adheres fairly well after the alcoholic base evaporates, and all of the oily or greasy bases tend to resist rinsing. You must take extra precautions when using a sunscreen with a lotion or cream base. Always remember to reapply it after swimming or perspiring heavily.

Under normal conditions, lipstick alone will protect the lips from all but the most intense sun-exposure. However, if your lips are thin, dry, or already damaged to some extent, supplementary protection may be indicated. Both Chapstick and Sea & Ski offer lip pomades containing amyl dimethyl PABA. Sun Stick is another brand that works well, and this uses digalloyl trioleate as the active ingredient.

On an individual basis, it has always been difficult to recommend one of the products giving a synthetic tan. This is because of the many variations in color that occur when these products are applied to different skins. The results may be indistinguishable from a natural tan or they may look completely phony. The chemical used to produce this tanning effect is dihydroxyacetone. It accomplishes this by imparting a stain to the dead cells of the skin's outer layer. Some people are afraid to use these products, thinking they might harm the skin, but they are perfectly safe. Remember, it is the real tan that always connotes sun damage, not the fake one. One product of this type that seems to give somewhat more predictable results is Sudden Tan, an aerosol. It also contains homosalate, a chemical sunscreen, and will furnish some protection. However, you should always apply this product very generously before exposure to direct sunlight.

The cleansing-products group includes the primary cleansers, such as soaps and rinsable cleansers, and the secondary cleansers, such as fresheners and medicated lotions. The medicated lotions differ in that they are capable of both cleansing and thinning skin.

The importance of having adequate information on each and every product you use has been stressed throughout this book. With most products, more usable information is continually being made available to the consumer. But soaps are an exception to this. Here, the situation is almost unbelievable. Soaps are not legally considered cosmetics and do not fall under the new labeling regulations. Consequently, the buyer has no legal right to know their composition or, more to the point, what she is using to cleanse her skin. The kindest way one can describe this piece of legislative idiocy is to call it an oversight. Like similar glaring errors in human judgment, it will probably be corrected in time. This would be of inestimable value to every consumer, who could then tell at a glance whether a cleansing bar was a true soap, a detergent, or a combination of the two. But for the present, this barrier to the evaluation of soaps remains. Legislation has been suggested that would require the listing of ingredients on household cleansing products. It would seem that the cleansers used on human beings deserve equal treatment, to say the least.

Always bear in mind that all bar soaps, regardless of composition, have a high irritant-potential for the human skin. With true soap, this is in part due to the elevated pH, or alkalinity. Detergents have a pH that is nearer neutral, but all of them have a predilection for attacking the skin's protein. In addition to the brands of true soaps already mentioned, Cashmere Bouquet and Jergens are perfectly acceptable for routine cleansing. As a rule, you should try to avoid the rather expensive soaps that are sold along with cosmetic lines. Most of these are superfatted—which means they are diluted with some noncleansing ingredient—so you don't even get 100 percent soap for your money, and these bars are often quite expensive. Most of them make better bath soaps than complexion soaps. Disregard the implications that any of these soaps can moisturize the skin, because this is physically impossible. In addition, the liquid soaps offered by cosmetic lines should likewise be avoided, since many of them contain detergents.

It is surprising how really few good rinsable cleansers there are on the market. The main trouble is that most of them lack rinsability. In addition, some are spiked with useless, noncleansing ingredients that do nothing but make the product more expensive. A properly formulated rinsable cleanser should rinse off easily and completely, with a minimum of rubbing, and should leave no trace of greasiness on your face. The rinsable lotions are preferable to the rinsable creams because they spread more easily, cleanse better, and rinse better. Super Skin is an alternate rinsable cleanser that seems to do a good job. Its main flaw is that it contains a large number of superfluous ingredients, but it seems to work well in spite of these. It is almost impossible to find a rinsable cleanser that is satisfactory in every respect, and recommending these products involves choosing the ones with the fewest deficiencies.

Never, never, under any circumstances, tissue off a rinsable cleanser and just let it go at that, even if this is what the label tells you to do. These labels are often written by people who don't know the facts, and they are frequently in error. Some people make the mistake of buying a product they think is a rinsable cleanser, only to find it doesn't rinse at all. You can avoid this mistake by insisting that the product you buy says "rinse-off" somewhere on the label. Furthermore, you should always avoid the rinsable creams and lotions that contain any type of medication. This can't possibly work in the minute or so the cleanser is in contact with the skin, and then everything goes down the drain. One highly advertised medicated rinsable cream started life many years ago as an insect-bite and sunburn remedy. Now, with hardly a mention of its shady past, it's being sold to the public as a complexion cleanser.

Most fresheners and medicated lotions are sold only as parts of cosmetic lines. This can often spell trouble for the consumer. Fresheners are also called toners, astringents, pore lotions, or skin tonics, but this doesn't in any way alter the character of these products. The only essential cleansing ingredient in either fresheners or medicated lotions is alcohol. This always was, and evermore shall be. With the exception of the chemical thinners found in medicated lotions, all of the other ingredients put into these cleansing products are at best useless, and at worst potentially harmful, to the skin.

You would think the cosmetic companies' insatiable demands for marketable novelties would be satisfied by the innumerable junk ingredients and chemical irritants used in many fresheners. (See Chapter VII.) But anyone who believes this has sadly underestimated their powers of imagination. For one thing, soaplike cleansing substances still appear in freshener formulas. If a freshener were used by itself, this might make some sense, but not when a soap is used beforehand. Many fresheners also contain MP ingredients. These are a complete waste if a regular MP film is applied after using them, as it should be. The eye-catching products that separate into two or more colored layers are usually of this type. Last on the list are the so-called "conditioners." In many instances, this term is an advertising euphemism for a humectant of some kind. These substances have the nasty habit of competing with the skin for moisture when the air is dry, so they are not to be trusted. Acceptable fresheners do exist in this jungle, but they are hard to find, and making your own still seems the best and safest course to follow. (See Chapter V.)

When buying a medicated lotion, always look at the label to be sure the product contains either salicylic acid or resorcin, because none of the other chemical thinners found in these products are strong enough to unclog the pores. The majority of prescriptions written for teenagers by dermatologists contains one or both of these ingredients. Antibacterial agents are often included in medicated lotions but, according to current theory, they are of little or no use to the adolescent skin. If the medicated lotion you are using doesn't seem to control the oiliness, try going over the skin with more than one saturated pad, possibly even three or four, and wiping more vigorously. If your medicated lotion seems ineffective in unclogging the pores, a larger amount should be patted on the skin at bedtime.

Of all the skin-care products, MP films probably show the greatest variations of both ingredients and prices. This is something of an anomaly because, in theory, they are the least complicated of products. The functional part of any MP film is always some water-impermeable substance, such as an oil, a grease, a wax, or any combination of these. The best MP films contain these three basic substances and nothing else. All of the heavier nighttime MP films mentioned in previous chapters correspond to this definition. It is important that heavy MP films be as free from irritants as possible, because they generally stay in intimate contact with the skin longer than any other type of product.

When the cosmetic chemist starts making these oils, greases, and waxes into lotions and creams, other things are added, and both the moisturizing ability and mildness of these products begin to decline, almost in direct proportion to the amount of extraneous material added. At the very least, both an emulsifying agent and a complete preservative system must be added to the basic MP ingredients to produce a lotion or cream. Normally, these are used as bases and worn under makeup during the day. The skin's salvation from these less agreeable lotions and creams lies in the fact that only very thin films are used, and they remain in place for relatively short periods of time. Other products of this type that are useful and generally kind to the skin include Lubriderm Lotion and Cream, and Keri Lotion and Cream. If one or more of the recommended daytime MP films doesn't suit you or function adequately as a makeup base, you might try these.

One of the greatest hoaxes ever perpetrated by the cosmetic industry is the claim that certain oils and greases of animal and vegetable origin moisturize better than those of mineral origin. Actually, a perusal of the scientific literature will show that the reverse is true. One excellent study* showed that light mineral oil and silicone oil caused a reduction in the moisture loss from human skin of 28 percent and 26 percent respectively, while oils of other origins managed a reduction ranging only from 23 percent to nil. Another swindle of almost equal frequency and importance is the endless variety of exotic and unusual ingredients, including humectants, that are put into MP products. Most of these are advertised as either increasing moisturization or conferring some other beneficial effect when, in fact, they either do nothing or decrease the product's moisturizing ability, sometimes by a considerable margin. For instance, the scientific study just mentioned showed that glycerine and propylene glycol, two favorite humectant substances, caused increases in moisture loss of 43 and 35 percent respectively.

Until recently, it was very difficult to identify the key ingredients in MP products, but the situation has changed considerably. According to a new Food and Drug Administration ruling, all cosmetic products must now have their ingredients listed on the label or package in order of decreasing predominance in the formula. This information greatly facilitates product comparisons, thereby helping consumers select products that are better suited to their individual needs. This means that the ingredient present in the greatest amount will be at the top of the list, while the

*D. H. Powers, and C. Fox, "A Study of the Effects of Cosmetic Ingredients, Creams and Lotions on the Rate of Moisture Loss from the Skin," *Proceedings of the Scientific Section of the Toilet Goods Association*, November 28, December 1957.

ingredient present in the least amount will be at the bottom. The new labeling regulations have other positive effects that should be of enormous benefit to the consumer, such as exposing the many ineffective and useless ingredients that hide behind trade names.

As an aid to using this information, lists of the more common MP ingredients found on product labels have been prepared. These ingredients have been divided into two basic groups, and classified as to whether or not they have moisturizing ability. With these lists, you will be able to tell by reading the product label which part of the formula is working for you and which is not. The relative positions of these ingredients in the product's qualitative formula should give you a fairly good idea of the overall moisturizing potential that lies within the tube or jar or bottle. Remember that these lists are by no means complete, and are intended only as a general guide:

MOISTURIZING INGREDIENTS

Greases

> Cocoa butter
> Hydrogenated oil
> Lanolin
> Petrolatum

Oils

> Avocado oil
> Butyl myristate or stearate
> Cod-liver oil

Cottonseed oil
Dimethicone
Grapeseed oil
Isopropyl palmitate or myristate
Mineral oil
Mink oil
Olive oil
Peach-kernel oil
Peanut oil
Pecan oil
Safflower oil
Shark-liver oil
Squalane
Turtle oil
Wheat germ oil

Waxes

Beeswax
Ceresin
Cetyl alcohol
Cetyl palmitate
Cholesterol
Glyceryl stearate
Microcrytalline wax
Paraffin
Propylene glycol stearate
Sorbitan stearate
Stearic acid
Stearyl alcohol

NON-MOISTURIZING INGREDIENTS

Allantoin
Aloe juice
Carrageenan
Cellulose gum
Egg
Estrogen
Gelatin
Glycerine
Hexalene glycol
Honey
Hydrolyzed animal protein
Milk
Pectin
PEG
Placenta extract
Poloxamer
PPG
Pregnenolone acetate
Progesterone
Propylene glycol
PVP
Royal jelly
Sorbitol
Urea
Vitamins
Yucca

The last entry on the list of nonmoisturizing ingredients, yucca, represents an almost perfect phonic expression of my emotional—and professional—reaction to most of the substances contained in this final list.

One of the happy consequences of good beauty care is that the women who practice it throughout life rarely need thinners, and those whose job it is to recommend these products are spared the frustrations of trying to find acceptable ones. The choice among abrasive thinners is limited, and most of them have various drawbacks. However, thinners are an indispensable beauty aid to most mature women, and a choice must be made. Although the abrasive surface thinners are somewhat easier on the skin than the abrasive particle thinners, equivalent amounts of dead skin theoretically can be removed with either, depending on the pressure applied and duration of the application. Consequently, this is another instance in which the user, rather than the manufacturer, determines the ultimate results. A new thinning product, a polyester sponge called Buf-Puf, has been recently introduced. The preliminary data furnished by the manufacturer are impressive, and this synthetic sponge may prove to be a worthy alternative to the loofa.

The main problems encountered with thinners are over-thinning, sometimes to the point where the skin is almost raw, and overcleansing. Problems of the latter type are not limited to the particle-type thinners having soap or detergent bases. Some of the surface-type thinners sold are accompanied by liquid cleansers. A specially textured cloth or mitten is usually part of the package, and the buyer is directed to use the two together. The cloth or mitten is fine, but the cleanser may contain a harsh detergent. Women of ancient Greece and Rome, who used almond meal and pumice, at least didn't have to contend with overcleansing problems.

Numerically speaking, makeup items form the cosmetic industry's largest group of products. This group is also the best as far as quality and value are concerned. Many dermatologists have for years recommended the Allercreme, Almay, and Marcelle lines of makeup, because these companies have always furnished dermatologists with the names of all the ingredients in their products. If a patient using these companies' makeup products developed an allergic reaction, the dermatologist, with immediate access to the various formulas, could more easily identify the offending ingredient. This information could also be very helpful in finding makeup for those known to be sensitive to specific ingredients. Nowadays, with all companies being required to disclose their ingredients, and the freedom from sensitizers being about equal among all popular brands, the reasons for recommending the makeup of these companies exclusively have disappeared. Furthermore, the word *hypoallergenic* has become meaningless, and companies that now use the term in their advertising may soon be forced by law to abandon it. Many dermatologists will continue to recommend Allercreme, Almay, and Marcelle products, not because they are "hypoallergenic," but because of a long tradition of service to the profession by the companies that make them.

Although the specific brand of makeup you wear can safely be left to your personal preference, there are a few things to be kept in mind while wearing it. Many makeup products do have ingredients that give them sunscreening and moisturizing ability, but makeup is designed to change your appearance, not improve the health of your skin. When you remove the makeup, you want the skin underneath to look at least as good as when you applied it. Unfortunately, this is not always the case, because makeup products are complex in nature, and their list of potential irritants is long. Pigments, powders, perfumes, dispersants, preservatives, humectants, antioxidants, alcohol, and alkalis are only a few

of the things with which your skin has to contend whenever
you apply makeup. Wear it if you must, for cosmetic
purposes, but don't be lulled into a false sense of security.

The beauty-service industry suffers from some of the
same maladies as the cosmetic industry. It, too, is backward
in many respects and shows similar variations in quality, the
services ranging from very beneficial to completely useless,
or in some cases even fraudulent. One bona fide excuse for
some of these shortcomings is that this is an industry of
independent agents, rather than large companies, and many
beauty operators are so poorly trained and have such limited
knowledge that they honestly don't know which of their
services are of value and which are not. More than likely,
the operator who sells you a useless service is less aware of
the larcenous nature of the transaction than, say, a cosmetic
company that sells you a useless product. The average
person would certainly tend to be more forgiving toward the
former than the latter if, indeed, forgiveness were extended
to either. A major contributing factor with regard to these
problems is the lack of uniform state and federal laws covering training, licensing, and regulation. There are certainly
good beauty schools, but there are also those that are un-
believably bad. On top of this, many operators receive the
bulk of their postgraduate education from cosmetic companies or the manufacturers of beauty equipment.

But the beauty-service field is a broad one, and the level
of competence of any individual operator becomes mean-
ingful only when considered in relation to the specific
services performed. On the average, it is hard to find fault
with the ethics and abilities of those operators who limit
themselves to hair and nail care. But when they also give
beauty treatments or facials, or perform these services
exclusively, the situation changes. It is in this area that we

find most of the beauty services of lower quality. Not only does much of it lack any demonstrable benefit, but some of these services may even be dangerous or harmful. Correction of the faults inherent in this part of the industry is hindered by the fact that local regulatory bodies often take the attitude that problems don't exist. The legal waters here are very murky, and the consumer generally receives little protection from either fraud or injury.

Some of the services rendered during the course of beauty treatments or facials are valuable and worth the cost, while others are not. As one might expect, most complete routines include services of both kinds. How do you tell the difference? Before trying to analyze specific procedures, it is necessary to separate the possible from the impossible, and see what can be done to the skin in sixty minutes or less that will realistically improve it. From a practical standpoint, there are only four general categories of beauty care that are known to benefit the human skin. These are environmental protection, moisturization, cleansing, and thinning. The first two can be eliminated immediately as not being adaptable to salon care, because of the conditions imposed by time and location. Outside of offering you refuge in the salon, an operator can obviously do nothing more with regard to environmental protection. As for moisturization, any MP film that might be applied during the course of a salon visit is rarely left in place more than five to ten minutes, a time insufficient for the film to have much effect on the skin's moisture level. This leaves cleansing and thinning, which are the only two theoretically useful services an operator can perform during the course of a visit. In other words, the only services any operator can offer that are both useful and capable of increasing beauty are those that remove something from the skin's surface. The things removed may be dirt, oil, dead cells, blackheads, hair, or any one of a number of undesirable substances. There is only one possible exception to this statement. Some beauty operators might contend that the various procedures that enlarge the small blood vessels of the skin, causing it to change color and swell slightly, are entirely legitimate. They might also argue that this is useful because it does cause a temporary improvement in the appearance, and doesn't do any harm if used in moderation. This phenomenon has previously been referred to as the "masque effect" and its many causes, both chemical and physical, are well known to beauty operators and widely used by them. In spite of arguments to the contrary, dermatologists have an essentially negative attitude toward the methods used to achieve this "masque effect."

The following is an analysis of some of the more popular procedures used in salons during the performance of beauty treatments or facials:

Useful Services

1. Cleansing with soap, rinsable cleanser, or alcoholic freshener.

2. Thinning the skin with motor-driven appliance, such as a rotating brush or other abrasive surface.

3. Removal of blackheads manually or with surgical instrument.

4. Removal of whiteheads or other small cysts with surgical instrument.

5. Thinning the skin, also known as "skin peeling" or "skin layering," with phenol, resorcin, trichloroacetic acid, enzymes, etc.

6. Temporary removal of superfluous hair by plucking, waxing, or the application of a chemical depilatory.

7. Permanent removal of superfluous hair by electrolysis.

Useless Services

1. Any manipulation placing the skin under physical stress, such as massaging, patting, kneading, rubbing, pulling or stretching, or the application of any vibrating appliance.

2. The application of wet or dry heat.

3. The application of cold in any form, including ice cubes or ice packs.

4. Any electrically operated wand, needle, plate, or ball, said to destroy bacteria, close or open the pores, remove any materials contained in the pores, prevent wrinkles, heal acne blemishes, or cause any substance, including water or animal serums, to pass into the skin.

5. Any vacuum or suction apparatus said to remove blackheads, dirt, or other débris from the skin's surface or pores.

6. Any electrically operated diagnostic equipment, said to give an indication of the skin's moisture level.

7. Any diagnostic test involving the removal of cells from the skin's surface, said to give an indication of the skin's moisture level, the size or contents of the pores, or the presence of deep wrinkles.

8. The insertion of an electric needle into the skin, said to allievate lines or wrinkles.

9. The use of diathermy, said to firm, thicken, or otherwise benefit the muscles of the face or neck.

10. The use of ultraviolet light, whether from a standard lamp or a glass rod or bulb of any shape, said to destroy bacteria.

11. The exposure to water-vapor mists, either hot or cold, said to promote a more rapid moisturization of the skin or open or close the pores.

12. The exposure to gases such as oxygen, carbon

dioxide, or ozone, said to sterilize the skin or improve its metabolism in any way.

13. The use of any bandage, wrapping, or strap, said to beneficially affect the skin or muscles.

14. The application of any masque, facial, or pack, said to promote moisturization, close or deep-cleanse the pores, or tighten or firm the skin.

15. The application of any electrical appliance that causes involuntary twitching of the muscles of the face or neck, said to stimulate these muscles.

An old friend who lives in another city called me recently He said that his wife, whom I had never met, was about to visit the salon of a cosmetologist who was famous for her flamboyant and unconventional approach to beauty care. My friend was concerned about the safety and efficacy of this beauty expert's methods, and wanted to know if I could offer any general advice on the subject.

I began by saying that, although his wife might benefit from a "skin peel," she would be well advised not to have it done by a cosmetologist. Otherwise, if she would avoid extreme heat and cold, anything that caused a sustained burning, cooling, or tingling sensation, anything that pulled or stretched the skin, and anything that was operated by electricity, with the exception of rotating brushes or electrolysis equipment, she would not only be safe from harm, but avoid practically all the outright frauds.

I haven't heard from my friend since that time, so I don't know what happened. I have a suspicion, however, that if his wife followed my advice to the letter, her visit to the cosmetologist's salon was one of the shortest on record.

X From a Dermatologist's Notebooks

This final chapter is a beauty miscellany containing facts, suggestions, and curiosities culled from notes accumulated over more than two decades. It includes a number of highly personal opinions, and I have also used it as a means of tying up some loose ends that were not securely knotted in previous chapters. If there is a beauty question that still puzzles you, the answer may very well be here. In any event, all of the items presented represent things that have struck me, at some time in the past, as being interesting enough to make a part of my permanent records.

I'VE GOT A SECRET

Did it ever occur to you that your best friend might have a tattoo hidden beneath her clothing? Although these are admittedly more common among men, the incidence of tattooed women is higher than you might think. The usual humdrum designs favored by men are also seen on women; however, the clandestine tattoos found on either the breasts or upper thighs of some women show considerable originali-

157

ty. The breasts are frequently inscribed with words of opposite meaning, like sweet and sour, hot and cold, chocolate and vanilla, etc. On the thighs, the tattoos often consist of an inscription alluding to some of the delights to be found in the vicinity. These are sometimes accompanied by arrows, presumably to guide those with a poor sense of direction. Tattoos are nearly always added by younger women, often under the influence of alcohol or drugs. If one of these tattooed women later marries someone with a restricted sense of humor, she will invariably want to have it removed. Unless the tattoo is large, this is a simple procedure and can be done by any plastic surgeon.

INSIDE JOB

Nothing applied externally can firm or tighten the skin. These qualities are determined solely by the skin's inner portion, and there is no cosmetic product or manipulation that has the least influence on this part of the skin.

SUPER MOISTURIZER

Cocoa butter is an excellent heavy MP film that can be purchased in any drug store. Since it is a waxy solid, melting it will greatly facilitate application. This can easily be accomplished by breaking a small piece off the bar and dropping it into a cup filled with hot water. After it liquefies, the cocoa butter will float as a film on the surface of the water and can be scooped up with the fingers.

CLOSE SHAVE

Many women who shave their legs develop a persistent

rash consisting of minute red "bumps" around the hair follicles. This is caused by the razor blade nicking the slightly raised follicular openings, but once it begins, it is usually made worse by soap. Problems of this sort can nearly always be solved by the dual approach of switching to an electric razor and trying not to shave too closely. Shaving the underarm area with a safety razor can cause the same difficulty, but here application of a deodorant immediately after shaving substantially increases the chances of irritating the skin or developing a rash.

BOOZE AND BEAUTY

There are few, if any, beautiful alcoholics. In addition to the internal damage done by large amounts of alcohol, many of these people also suffer from various nutritional problems, including vitamin deficiencies. The combination of the two is enough to erase any beauty a woman might once have possessed.

HELP FOR SHIPWRECKED HAIR

Hot oil treatments are the living fossils of the hair care field. This is not to say they are completely useless, because all oils have some conditioning effect on the hair. It's just that modern conditioners work so much better in every respect. However, if you are stranded on a desert island with a head of sick hair, applying coconut oil or any other readily available vegetable oil would be a very helpful form of first aid.

SEXUAL EQUALITY AND MAKEUP

Does painting the face play into the hands of male chauvinists? Is makeup dehumanizing? Is it a handicap in the struggle for sexual equality? Put another way, if both sexes used makeup, and the man in your life suddenly began wearing lipstick, foundation, blusher, mascara, and eyeshadow, would it make him more or less attractive to you? If your answer is less, than you must ask yourself why it should make you any more attractive to him.

CLUES TO LONGEVITY

It has been shown experimentally that rats not only remain healthier, but live longer, if they are fed the minimum number of calories necessary to sustain life, kept in a cool environment, and not allowed to overexert themselves. Theoretically, a skinny, cold rat that slept a lot could live forever. Human beings might do well to emulate these experimental rodents.

PROBLEM TOENAILS

Stories about sick toenails don't often move the listener to tears, but even these prosaic appendages have their problems. The two most common are ingrown toenails and separation of the nails from their beds. Not only is an ingrown toenail uncomfortable, but it may eventually penetrate the skin, paving the way for a severe infection. This can usually be prevented if small balls or wisps of cotton are kept pushed under the lateral edge of the ingrown nail near the corner, using a toothpick or other small instrument. This elevates the sharp edge of the nail and encourages it to grow outward, instead of down into the flesh. If this is not successful, then the lateral edge and corner of the nail should be clipped as closely as possible. As a last resort, there is a minor surgical operation that will permanently remove the ingrown section of the nail. Although separated toenails may result from a fungus infection or thyroid problem, in most instances the cause is strictly mechanical in origin. The only remedies are keeping the nails short and wearing loose-fitting shoes with low heels.

GIBBERISH

Why do some beauty writers insist on using vague and inaccurate terms when more precise ones are ready and waiting? A good example is the verb *refine,* which appears frequently in the cosmetic literature. Someone or other is always "refining" the skin or "refining" the pores. The dictionary defines this word as "to free from impurities." Why, then, don't they just say *cleanse?* The word *tone* is abused in a similar fashion, and is often used in ways that defy rational interpretation. In my opinion, *tone* should be stricken from the beauty vocabulary, and its use limited to discussions involving music.

SECRETARY SPREAD

A woman who sits at a desk all day is likely to blame her job when she finds that her posterior is getting progressively larger and losing its shape. But this is not entirely fair, because bottoms were made to be sat upon, and are not normally enlarged or deformed by doing so. The secretaries who complain most loudly are usually those who keep snacks in their desks, and have an almost religious conviction against any form of regular exercise. Secretary spread is not an occupational problem: it is a fat problem, caused by too many calories and too little exercise.

ALL ABOUT pH

You've probably heard about pH, which refers to acid-alkaline balance. The living skin seems to prefer a neutral or slightly acid pH that is between 5.0 and 6.0, the average among women being about 5.5. The hair, being dead, doesn't care. However, many cosmetic products are sold on the basis of their pH. Is this just another gimmick, or is there something to it? The answer is that it is often used as a gimmick but, under certain circumstances, there is definitely something to it. The situation differs according to whether we are talking about the skin or the hair. As a rule, if a product stays in contact with the skin longer than a few minutes, as do MP films, sunscreens, and makeup, a neutral pH is very desirable. If the product is in contact with the skin for only a brief period, such as cleansers and thinners are, a neutral pH is desirable, but not essential. This is because the skin has, within limits, the ability to adjust its own pH. For instance, all true soaps are alkaline, and the skin surface becomes alkaline after using them, but the healthy skin can bring itself back to neutral in a very short time. The hair is different, in that it can tolerate mild alkalinity for long periods. Of the three best-selling shampoos, Head and Shoulders and Prell are moderately alkaline and Johnson's Baby Shampoo is mildly alkaline. This would seem to indicate that healthy hair is not harmed by the regular use of a product having a higher pH. On the other hand, if you are using a shampoo containing a hair-conditioner, the pH may be very important, since it will often determine how much of the conditioner sticks to the hair shaft. With this exception, any allusion to the pH of a shampoo or other hair-care product can be safely ignored.

HAIRY ILLUSION

Shaving doesn't make hair any coarser or increase the number of actively growing hairs. It just seems that way, because a short stubble feels coarser to the touch than a growth of longer hairs, and this also tends to reinforce the impression that more hairs are present than there actually are.

METABOLIC MYTH

Even though we are rapidly approaching the twenty-first century, there are still rational and otherwise intelligent people who cling to the belief that the skin "breathes." These people are in error, because the skin doesn't take oxygen directly from the air but depends on the lungs to do this for it. In accordance with the usual workings of human physiology, the skin receives oxygen and discharges wastes through the small blood vessels. Under no circumstances does the body ever "breathe" through the skin, and the skin certainly doesn't need direct access to the atmosphere, or ever "breathe" independently. You can better appreciate this if you will visualize someone who has broken a bone and been in a cast for some weeks or months. When the cast is removed, the skin, far from having succumbed to asphyxiation, looks fine. Obviously, being confined by an air-tight cast hasn't hurt it at all. In some ways, it looks even better than before. This is because the skin has been protected from the environment and has enjoyed a moisture level close to 100 percent during the time the cast was in place.

Although the skin does many fascinating things, breathing is not among them.

MORE ABOUT MOLES

The small, elevated red spots that sometimes start during pregnancy, and appear in great profusion on older people, are called *angiofibroma*. These are a type of mole and they are always benign. Removing them is unnecessary unless one becomes irritated by the clothing or grows large enough to create a cosmetic problem.

CONFUSED CRUSADERS

The consumer advocates who spend most of their time questioning the safety of cosmetic products may be doing the public a disservice, as well as playing into the hands of the cosmetic companies, which are delighted to have attention focused on the safety question. This is because there is no safety problem of any real consequence. To substantiate the claim that cosmetics are relatively safe, there is the fact that, during 1973, the Food and Drug Administration averaged only about two letters of complaint a day. The actual number of reactions or injuries from cosmetic products is estimated at about ten thousand per year. This means that only about one person out of twenty thousand has trouble with a cosmetic product during the course of a year. Certainly, the incidence of reactions to things like strawberries or shellfish is a great deal higher. The real problems lie in the areas of ineffective products and consumer frauds.

MOCK TURTLE

I once knew a chemist who worked for a company that

made several highly advertised products containing turtle oil. This is a relatively expensive oil, and you wouldn't expect to find a high percentage of it in any cosmetic product—in this specific instance, the amounts used were minuscule. When the turtle oil was added to a batch during the manufacturing process, the chemist referred to it as "running the turtle through the tank." When he told me this story, I immediately conjured up a mental picture of one of the small turtles sold at pet stores, tied to a string, being gingerly lowered into a huge tank for a few seconds, and then quickly retrieved. As a matter of fact, there is a movement under way to ban the cosmetic use of turtle oil altogether. This is a conservation measure designed to save the sea turtle. Since turtle oil has no unique properties, it certainly wouldn't be missed.

MAKEUP FOR BLACK SKIN

Black women often find that makeup designed for lighter skins is not suitable for them, since it seems to turn shades of orange or pink on darker skins, or give it a gray cast. Now there are makeups designed specifically for the black skin, and black women have benefited from the general trend toward lighter, more transparent makeups. The new gel products adapt well to dark skin of almost any shade.

PLAYING IT COOL

The recent energy crisis produced some unexpected, and probably unappreciated, beauty bonuses. Lowering the temperature of the living quarters during winter results in a skin that is not only more moist, but more attractive. As far as beauty is concerned, warm is ugly and cool is beautiful.

THE FTC AND FDA

When a woman is disappointed with a cosmetic product for some reason or other, she often blames the Federal Trade Commission for not suppressing the deceptive advertising that induced her to buy it, or the Food and Drug Administration for not telling her the product was ineffective before she bought it. But these federal agencies are not necessarily to blame. They only carry out the laws made by your representatives in Congress, and often don't have the legal right to do anything about either situation. Even in cases where they are authorized to take action, they may not have sufficient money or manpower to enforce the law. Therefore, the blame should be placed squarely on your representatives in Congress, who make the laws these regulatory bodies have to obey and approve the fiscal appropriations they need to do their work. Nevertheless, if you think you have been misled or defrauded, by all means file a complaint with the Federal Trade commission. Every regional office has forms for this purpose but, due to lack of jurisdiction, manpower, or both, they may be able to give you very little satisfaction.

If you think there is something wrong with the product itself, write the Food and Drug Administration. It is eager to have these reports and will keep yours for reference, but may be similarly powerless to investigate or remedy the situation.

Both agencies are now awaiting new laws that will give them the muscle to combat some of the problems now prevalent in the beauty business. Your representatives are the only ones who can authorize these things, so let them know your wishes. The drug and cosmetic industry has been making its wishes known in Washington for years, and the fact that these are always accompanied by large political contributions may make them seem more reasonable than yours. This particular industry is very high on the list of big givers, and this is one reason why it has never been under much pressure to mend its ways. So if the consumer doesn't speak up, things are probably going to continue pretty much as they have in the past.

SUNTAN SUBSTITUTES

Many people won't use the products that stain the skin to simulate tanning, because they are afraid that freckles or other pigment spots will become more noticeable. These products don't increase the skin's natural pigment, but impart a uniform stain to the surface, so apprehensions regarding these undesirable effects are groundless.

FACIAL EXERCISES AND MASSAGE

Facial exercises are not only a waste of time, but may actually harm the skin. To increase the thickness of the facial muscles enough to cause any noticeable plumping effect on the skin, you would theoretically have to do these exercises twenty-four hours a day for the rest of your life. Think how many pushups it would take to increase the diameter of your biceps by just one-eighth inch! If you have damaged skin, all of this pulling and stretching can further weaken the tissues and increase wrinkling and sagging, instead of helping it. I once heard an advocate of these exercises tell someone that chin muscles could be "toned" by trying to touch the tip of the nose with the tongue twenty times a day. However, the only possible result of this is a longer tongue. If you are already doing this exercise, be sure to stop before the

tongue gets too long to fit comfortably back into the mouth.
Along these same lines, massaging the face or neck may also
weaken the skin if it is done too vigorously.

HIGH-ALTITIUDE HAZARDS

A note to the ski enthusiasts: sun intensity increases about
20 percent for every thousand meters of elevation. For
instance, if you were going to ski from the top of Mount
Everest, and remain adequately protected, you would have
to triple the strength of your sea-level sunscreen.

COSMETIC APPLIANCES

There seems to be a revival of interest in chin-straps. The
only thing these do is keep fluid from accumulating in the
loose tissues of the neck when you are lying down. Even
without a chin-strap, the pull of gravity will remove this
excess fluid shortly after you arise in the morning.

Apropos of this, a woman can now retire for the night
looking like an accident victim who has just left the operating room. There are masks made of a special material that
are supposed to massage and increase the "tone" of the facial
muscles, and gloves of the same material that are supposed
to make the nails grow by increasing circulation. Both of
these are worthless, of course.

PIGMENT LOSS

Vitiligo is a condition in which the skin pigment disappears. It is not actually a disease, because the skin remains
normal in every other respect. Sometimes the pigment
returns, and sometimes it doesn't. At present, there is no
really effective treatment for vitiligo.

BEAUTY-CONTEST WINNER

If you are over forty and would like a graphic demonstration of what environmental protection can do, mark off a square inch on your cheek, then a square inch on a part of your hip that would normally be covered by clothing or a bathing suit. Then compare these areas with the aid of a mirror. You will see remarkable differences in texture, color, and contour. The results will probably make you wish you could trade the tired-looking stuff on your face for the more attractive skin on your hip.

PRODUCT PERFORMANCE DATA

It is technically possible to give consumers a great deal more helpful information about beauty products than they are now receiving. Studies showing the relative protection offered by uniform films of sunscreens are commonplace in the scientific literature. These evaluations could be standardized, extended to all commercial sunscreens, and the relative efficiency of each individual product noted on its label. It is also possible to express a skin cleanser's relative mildness of harshness by means of a numerical value, as well as its ability to remove dirt. Various moisturizers can also be compared with regard to their effectiveness in retarding the evaporation of water from the skin's surface. In many instances, the appearance of this information on product labels would be very helpful.

READING BETWEEN THE LINES

I am constantly amazed at the deviousness of some cosmetic advertising. A good example is the promotion of collagen protein as an ingredient in skin care products. One technique used is the apposition of two true statements which, when taken together, are supposed to create a false impression in the buyer's mind. The advertisement usually begins by saying that collagen protein is the main constituent of firm, young skin, which is true, and that the product being advertised contains this substance, which is also true. There is no further explanation, and the workings of the reader's imagination are expected to make the sale. These two statements give the impression that the collagen protein in the product has the ability to replace aging and damaged collagen in human skin, which is not true.

What these advertisements don't point out is that the collagen protein in the product is of animal origin, that it's dead as a doornail, that it can't penetrate the skin, and that even if it did, it couldn't in any way replace living human collagen or be of any help in preventing wrinkling or sagging. Advertisements like this are, in many ways, just as dishonest as picking pockets or holding up liquor stores.

EMERGENCY CALL

A surprising number of the emergency calls received by dermatologists concern sunburn. The victim has usually stayed out in the sun too long on one of the first warm, sunny days of summer, or fallen asleep under a sunlamp. Once the damage is done, all the sufferer can do is soak in a cool tub of water, apply a little baby oil to the skin afterward, and take aspirin for pain. The anesthetic sprays advertised for sunburn do give relief, but they often cause allergies and are best avoided.

HOOEY, HUNGARY STYLE

There is a company that sells a line of cosmetic products

formulated with water imported from Hungary. The theory is that Hungarian women owe their legendary beauty to the magnesium contained in their drinking water, and that products made with this water are superior in some way. If this were true, the women residing in certain counties of Texas would be absolutely ravishing, as the mineral content of the local water is extremely high. As it is, however, the beauty assets of these women are only average.

FIRST AID

The best treatment for minor cuts, scratches, or abrasions is to wash the affected area twice a day with plain soap and water and apply a plastic bandage. However, this bandage should always be removed and the area left uncovered during the night. The people who make these little dressings may not agree with this, but they are in the business of selling as many as possible. If a hard scab develops, a little petrolatum or Vaseline may be applied at bedtime. Iodine or other strong antiseptics should never be used on these wounds.

SUNBURN AND WIND

It has recently been shown that sunburn is intensified by wind. This means that you should always use a sunscreen with a moisturizing base if the day is windy.

BEAUTY BEHIND BARS

A short time ago, while participating in a group discussion, I learned that the man sitting next to me had just finished serving a fifteen-year sentence for manslaughter. After overcoming the initial apprehension one might feel in sitting next to such a man, I relaxed and thoroughly enjoyed talking with him. Although middle-aged, his appearance struck me as being exceptionally youthful and trim. I then realized that for the past fifteen years, he had enjoyed a high degree of environmental protection, courtesy of the state in which he was incarcerated and, with prison food being what it is, probably had little opportunity to get fat during his stay. This isolated incident proves nothing, of course, but it would be fascinating to study the inmates of a women's prison and see how those who have spent many years behind bars compare with their contemporaries on the outside.

USELESS DUPLICATION

One of the most unnecessary things on earth is the production of different kinds of moisturizers for areas that are separated physically but covered with skin of a similar thickness. The existence of both eye and throat moisturizers is an example of this.

CONTROVERSIAL HORMONE

One ploy widely used by the cosmetic industry to sell products is to loudly proclaim that something is different from what it obviously is. I once had an argument with a cosmetic company executive about an ingredient used in one of his products, which he claimed was a "nonhormone." He defended this classification by saying that the substance in question was synthetic and not to be found among the hormones that occur naturally in the human body. I countered by saying that its chemical structure looked suspiciously like that of a hormone, and the effects on the skin were almost identical to those caused by hormones. If it barks, has fleas, and fetches the newspaper, it's a dog, to my way of thinking, no matter what anyone calls it.

STRESS VERSUS ALLERGY

People often have the impression that many of the skin problems treated by dermatologists are caused by nervousness. If this were true, the incidence of these problems among those in mental institutions would be extremely high, but this is not the case. Actually, one of the few skin problems that occurs in response to mental stress is hives, or urticaria. You may have noticed, at one time or another, the blotchy, red eruption that will appear occasionally on the neck and chest of a young girl when she is subjected to stress, such as being introduced to someone of the opposite sex whom she finds highly attractive, or a luminary of some sort who makes her feel ill at ease. This condition is closely related to hives. Other more severe forms of this abnormality often involve the entire body. In many cases, allergies such as those to medications, foods, or inhalants play a part. Hives is usually treated by allergists, rather than dermatologists. As a rule of thumb, dermatologists treat allergies of external origin, such as those to cosmetics, while those of internal origin are in the realm of the allergist.

HAND-PROTECTION

There are a number of protective creams sold for use by women with "housewife's hands." I have never found one that works very well—certainly not as well as rubber gloves worn in the proper manner.

SMOKING AND WRINKLES

Someone concluded a few years ago that there was a definite correlation between smoking and wrinkles. As often happens in the field of scientific research, another investigator made a similar study and came to the opposite conclusion. If the past is any guide, there may be several more investigations giving conflicting results before something is proved conclusively one way or the other. It would be difficult to adequately control a study like this, due to the many mental and physical differences between smokers and nonsmokers. It is likely that the cigarette will eventually prove to be a symptom, rather than a cause.

EMBEDDED WHITEHEADS

It is almost impossible to remove whiteheads by any method that doesn't pierce the skin, such as surgical extraction with the point of a scalpel, or burning with an electric needle. This is invariably true in the case of older skin. In adolescents, the vigorous use of an abrasive cleanser can sometimes remove a few of the smaller whiteheads.

SKIN SPIDERS

The enlarged blood vessels that appear as minute red blotches are colloquially known as "spiders," because individual lesions consist of a large central vessel, fed by several subsidiary vessels that resemble legs. This arrangement can easily be seen with the aid of a magnifying glass. Dermatologists treat these lesions, but the central vessel must be obliterated to dispose of the "spider," and this is sometimes difficult to do.

UGLY SCARS

Thick scars in prominent locations, due to injuries or surgical operations, can be major beauty handicaps. Some scars will show a considerable decrease in thickness over a period of months or years, but others seem to remain static. Injecting cortisone directly into the scar is often helpful. In other cases, excision of the scar, followed by X-ray treatments, gives good results.

TROUBLESOME TAGS

The small moles that seem to be attached to the skin by short stalks are called "skin tags." The necks of some women become almost covered with these small growths, especially during middle age and the later years. They are easy to remove, but new ones keep appearing. Fortunately, they are always benign.

SILICONE INJECTIONS

Women continue to submit to silicone injections, even though the Food and Drug Administration has stipulated that this fluid be used only for investigational purposes. (Therefore, any unauthorized injection is illegal.) Silicone is injected directly into breasts to enlarge them, and also into wrinkles and lines, where its plumping action compensates for underlying tissue loss. The danger lies in droplets of this fluid leaving the injection site and entering the general circulation. These have been found in the brain, liver, and other internal organs. The injection of silicone fluid is vastly different from silicone breast implants, which are made by encapsulating the fluid in a nontoxic, nonabsorbable container. These are used to enlarge undersized breasts, and are absolutely safe. With these implants in place, any flat-chested woman can be the equal of her better-endowed sisters.

MISPLACED MOISTURIZERS

You will occasionally see advertisements claiming a certain moisturizing ingredient is superior because it penetrates the skin. However, evidence that any moisturizing ingredient can pass through the skin in substantial quantities has never appeared in any reputable scientific journal. The studies purporting to show this are usually done under the aegis of some cosmetic company to demonstrate the advantages of a particular ingredient or product. You can always hire someone to prove that the sun rises in the west and sets in the east, but this sort of thing is neither scientifically nor morally acceptable. It doesn't really make any difference, however, because if moisturizers did penetrate the skin, they wouldn't do much good circulating around inside the body, not to mention the ill effects this would cause. Moisturizers should always be on top of the skin, where moisture is escaping, rather than somewhere beneath it.

DANGER SIGNAL

The unattractive yellow plaques that appear on the eyelids of mature women are called *xanthomas*. In some cases, they are associated with an elevated blood cholesterol; in others, there is no internal abnormality of any kind. The lesions themselves can easily be removed by a physician, but they tend to recur.

NOTE FROM EUROPE

During the early part of my career, I worked in hospitals in both England and France, and so was able to observe the beauty characteristics of the populations at first hand. One thing I noticed was that English women had much better complexions than their French counterparts just across the Channel. I'm sure part of the explanation lies in the quality of beauty care prevalent in each country. The English women don't necessarily do anything out of the ordinary; it's just that the French seem to have originated most of the wrong approaches to beauty care. They have exported these concepts all over the world, and now the chicken-embryo serum, placental extract, and all the rest of this voodoo is coming back to haunt them.

SKIN HEMORRHAGES

Older women often notice the appearance of dusky red spots, sometimes up to an inch in diameter, on the forearms. These are caused by broken blood vessels in the skin, and usually follow bruising, pinching, or some other minor injury. This is often so insignificant that the older person is unaware it has happened. Sometimes internal diseases contribute to this problem, but usually the person is healthy and the fault lies entirely with the blood vessels themselves, which are so weak and fragile that they break in response to the slightest strain. Hemorrhages of this sort are often treated with Vitamin C, but successful results are rare. The only remedy lies in being as careful as possible.

WATER AND WEIGHT CONTROL

Many obese women think they can lose weight effortlessly by raising the skin's temperature in steam baths or saunas. This activates the sweat glands, and weight is lost, but it is all in the form of water, not fat. After boiling their bodies for an hour or so, these women drink several glasses of water, and back comes the weight. Silly, isn't it? The practice of body wrapping has a similar effect.

PLENTIFUL INGREDIENT

When a friend of mine in the cosmetic business finally realized that water is the only thing that softens the skin, he conceived the idea of improving one of his moisturizing products by increasing the water content. I tried to dissuade him from this, pointing out that additional ingredients were needed in the product to seal in the moisture. As ridiculous as this dialogue may sound, some companies seem to formulate their moisturizing products according to this line of reasoning. This is why some moisturizing lotions and creams are very much like the bottom of a boat—close to 100 percent water!

PRIZE POSSESSION

Many young women seem to value a new nose above almost anything else in the world. A plastic surgeon can literally remake a nose to order: taking out a hump, shortening the nose, reshaping the nostrils, or even building up a saddle nose. This operation is one of the simplest and least traumatic of all the plastic procedures, and can be done any time after bone growth is completed. The recipients of nose jobs always experience a much greater psychologic boost than the degree of change would seem to warrant. Noses, apparently, have a mystique all their own.

TEMPORARY LIFT

The headbands that temporarily decrease the depth of wrinkles by stretching the skin do cause a modest improvement in the appearance, and apparently do no harm. The amount of tension produced by such appliances is slight, much less than that caused by facial massage or the other things that pull or stretch the skin. This is analogous to shaping the figure by wearing a bra or girdle. These temporary lifts go back to the beginning of history, and it has often been a question of fashion whether to support the tissues of the face and figure, or allow them to seek their own level.

BOOBY PRIZE

The prize for imaginative copy in the beauty field should go to the writer at a leading fashion magazine who, in recommending a skin cream containing collagen protein, described its action as " 'threading' elastic through those tired out pores." Even the thought of such a thing boggles the mind.

DIRTY TRICK

In some salons, a so-called peeling lotion is applied during the course of beauty treatments or facials that supposedly removes dead skin. The operator massages the lotion into the face until small balls appear, which are then wiped away, and the customer breathes a sigh of relief upon seeing the huge quantity of dead skin that this miracle of modern beauty care has removed from her exterior. But, wait a minute! The little balls are not composed of dead skin, but dried solids derived from the lotion itself. Products having this particular characteristic are called "roll-ball" lotions in the trade, a most appropriate name.

AN APOLOGY

During the course of my scientific writings over the years, I have drawn conclusions from personal observations and expressed opinions that I believe to be correct. But some of these will eventually prove to be wrong, and I sincerely hope that anyone who has a contrary opinion will try to show me where I may have gone astray. If there is a better approach to beauty care, I am as eager to learn about it as anyone. In any field of science, truth is ascertained only by a process of continually testing different ideas by pitting one against the other. This is why I don't mind in the least if someone tries to refute one of my ideas. It shows that my opponent is thinking and, when people on opposite sides of a question do this, progress toward the truth is inevitable.

Index